Air Fryer for Two Cookbook

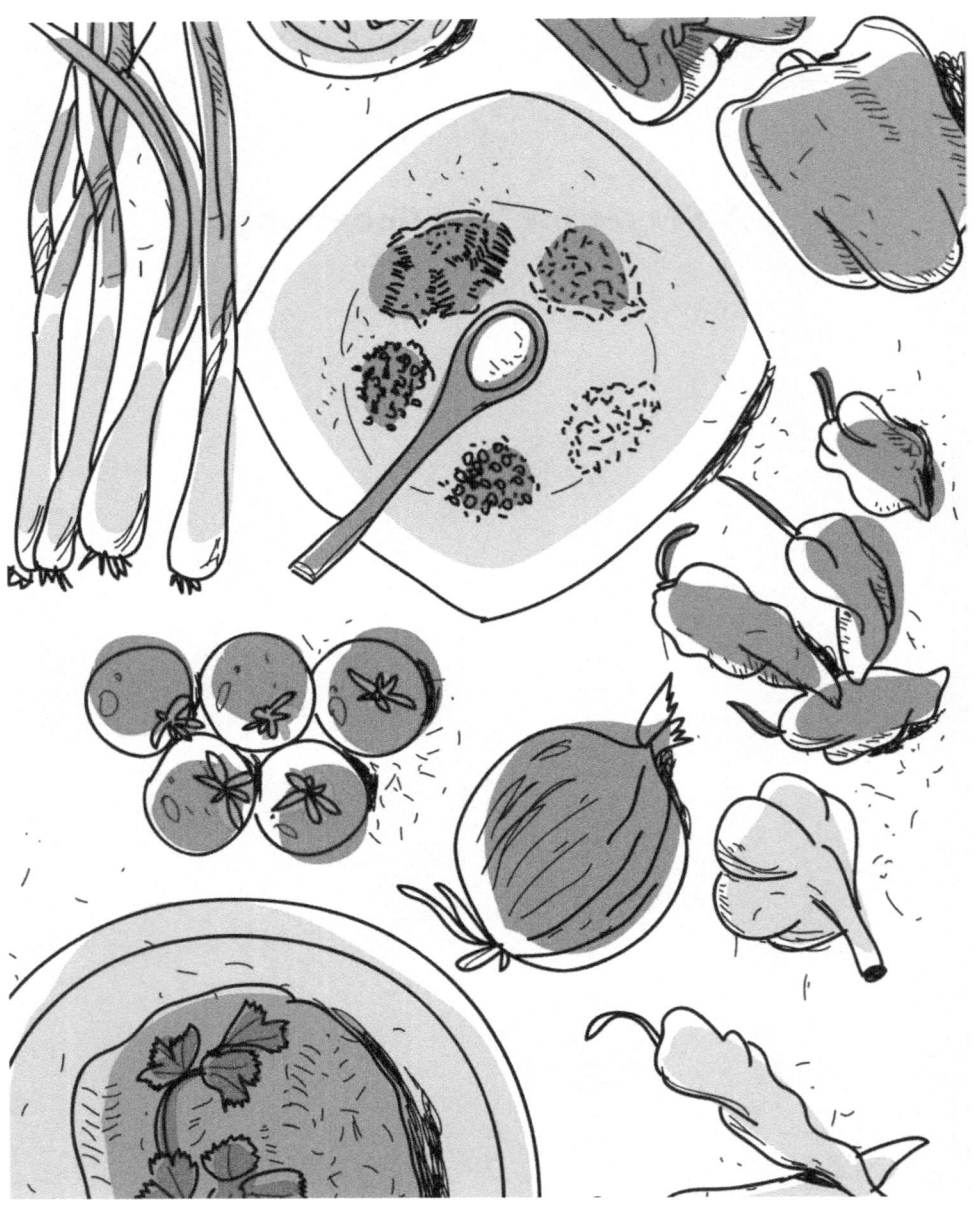

Air Fryer
for Two
Cookbook

Air Fryer Recipes for Two People
to Enjoy Together

Brenda Gilbert

"For my family, to whom I owe my daily happiness and love for life and food."

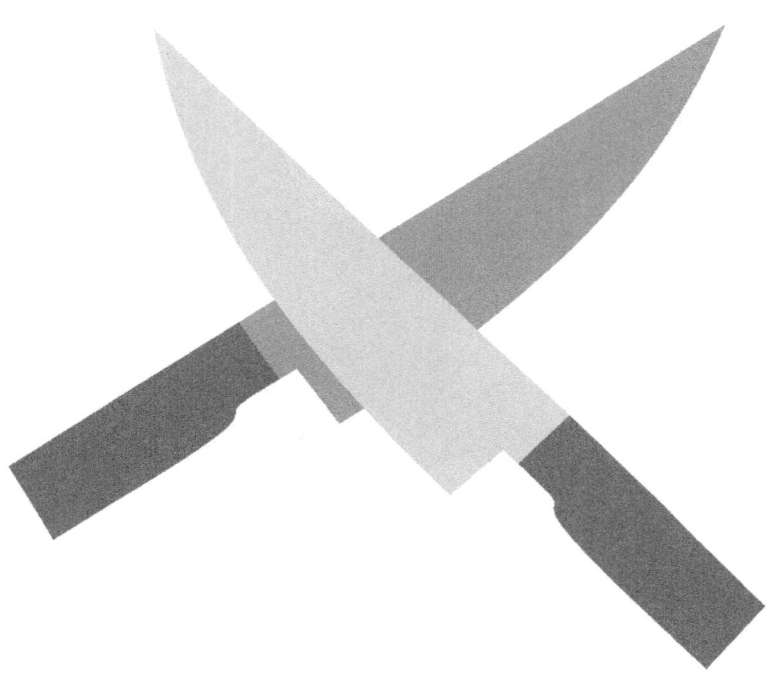

TABLE OF CONTENTS

Author Avatar

Several years ago I noticed that everyone I knew was suddenly talking about air fryers. At first I assumed it would be a passing trend and my friends' air fryers would end up gathering dust in their cupboards. However, they kept using them, and when I tasted the chicken wings and zucchini chips my best friend prepared with hers, I decided to seriously consider buying one of my own. When I started looking through buying guides, I was thoroughly impressed. There were so many to choose from! Philips may have created the first air fryer, but now there are brands from Cuisinart and T-fal Actifry. It's just me and my partner at home, so I didn't need the biggest size, but I did want to be able to cook larger food items. I ended up getting a 6-quart model, just to be safe. My friends were making dishes and snacks like cakes and pizza, and a 6-quart was able to fit the necessary accessories. I also decided on getting a model with temperature controls on a digital display. There isn't anything wrong with analog, but I like being really precise when it comes to heat. I don't have the sharpest instincts when it comes to cooking food perfectly, so I like to have appliances that do the work for me.

Once I had my air fryer, it was time to cook. I started out simple first with French fries and then with the zucchini chip recipe from my friend. The French fries tasted better than what I could get at some fast food restaurants! The zucchini chips were also great, especially when seasoned with salt, pepper, garlic, and a little paprika.

Since that day years ago when I first opened the box and set up the fryer, we've made all kinds of veggie fries and chips (sweet potato fries, kale chips, cauliflower bites), chicken wings, fish 'n chips, mini cinnamon rolls, and even homemade pop tarts.

It's been tempting to just make a lot of my junk food favorites all day every day, but I know that even air-fried onion rings are still, at the end of the day, onion rings. I've made it a goal to prepare lots of veggie recipes in my air fryer. My partner and I are eating way more vegetables than we did in the past and I can see the positive results. The air fryer is just so convenient and the veggies taste better than the usual steamed variety. I don't feel like I'm forcing myself to eat something I don't really like just because it's healthy. We buy so many fresh veggies now that we know just about everyone down at our local farmer's market.

I'm not usually one to jump on any bandwagon, but I'm really glad I got on board with the air fryer. After seeing the wide variety of foods my friends were making, I knew this gadget wasn't just some gimmick. Having owned and used one myself for years, it's become my favorite appliance. It's easy to use, easy to clean, and I depend on it for quick, healthy meals and for party food that isn't exactly "healthy," but that's healthier than deep-frying. Everyone needs to treat themselves. The air fryer lets me do that guilt-free.

I hope you, your family, and your friends enjoy these recipes. Whether you are eating to lose weight and cut out unhealthy oil, or just because you love the taste, there is something here for you.

Enjoy!
Brenda Gilbert

Introduction

Air fryers are all the rage these days with notable chefs like Gordon Ramsey singing their praises. What is an air fryer exactly? Why is it special? This introduction breaks down the why and how of air fryers as well as the benefits and downsides every buyer should be aware of. When used correctly to cook certain foods, an air fryer can be a great addition to a healthy kitchen. You'll learn how to choose the one that's best for you, as well as the process of using it. Air fryers are very easy to cook with and can make everything from French toast sticks to egg rolls. After using your air fryer, you want to keep it clean and well-cared for, so we've included cleaning tips, soap recommendations, and tips on troubleshooting any problems. The last section runs through the best advice from blogs and brands so you can make delicious meals in your air fryer for years to come.

I. AIR FRYERS 101

The air fryer as we know it came from Philips. They gave their product a simple name: The Air Fryer. The big claim of this new gadget was that it could fry food using 80% less fat than traditional deep-fryers. The air fryer became an overnight success in the United States, as well as countries like Japan and Australia. You can now find air fryers from a variety of brands all claiming to perform better or just as good as the Philips.

What is an air fryer exactly? How do they work? Air fryers work like convection ovens, which means they circulate hot air around an enclosed chamber to cook food. There are a lot more styles of air fryers than convection ovens, however, and many models are significantly cheaper. An air fryer is made of just a few parts: a heating element, fan, and cooking chamber.

The heating element, which sits above the cooking chamber and food, will most likely reach around 400-degrees. A fan circulates that hot air around the chamber, enveloping food in a blanket of consistent heat, so everything cooks evenly. This produces what's known as the Maillard Reaction, which is essentially the reason for why cooked, browned food tastes so good. Heat transforms sugars, proteins, and more into a new, delicious form.

If you get a Philips air fryer, it will be equipped with their patented Rapid Air Technology, which is known for its speed and effectiveness. On all brands, the fryer's cooking chamber can be pulled out like a drawer for easy cleaning. Most also come with a food separator. You do *not* put oil in the cooking chamber; the food is coated before it goes inside the fryer. To prevent too much heat from building pressure, the fryer will also have some kind of exhaust system.

Air fryers use superheated air, a fan, and cooling system to fry food using 80% less oil than a deep fryer. Thanks to the Maillard Reaction, food gets crispy and delicious.

Other than the three main parts, air fryers will also have a timer and a way to adjust the temperature, like a knob or digital display. Some will also come with presets for foods like French fries, potato chips, steak, and so on. Digital units tend to cost more because they're more precise.

Basket vs. paddle air fryers

There are two types of air fryers you can choose from. Basket air fryers are the most common and easy to use. They get the "basket" part of their name because that's where you put the food. During the frying process, you have to shake that basket a few times to guarantee evenly-cooked food. On the plus side, they are very affordable.

Paddle air fryers are built with a self-stirring paddle, so no shaking is required. The other benefit is you can make dishes like curry and risotto. You do need to put a bit more oil on the food, and the paddle fryers are more expensive than the basket type.

So, should you get a basket or paddle air fryer? It all depends on what you want to cook and how much money you're willing to spend. If you don't care about shaking the basket a few times and you don't plan on making more liquidy dishes, go with a basket air fryer because they are more affordable.

Benefits of air-frying

It seems like everyone is talking about air fryers, but why? Why makes them so great? There are five main reasons motivating customers to buy this specialized kitchen appliance:

Speed

Food cooks really quickly when it's air-fried. It takes less time to cook in an air fryer compared to an oven, stovetop, or deep fryer. Homemade French fries (made with fresh potatoes) take just 20 minutes, while raw meatballs are done in around 10 minutes. Reheating food is also much faster because of the high temperatures. Also, unlike food heated back up in the microwave, it doesn't end up soggy. Making a meal for just two people can be done in a snap, and if you need to do multiple batches when you have people over, each batch doesn't take a lot of time.

Ease of use

Using a deep fryer can be tricky because you have to watch the temperature of the oil. Air fryers are much easier because you just set the temp on the unit itself and wait for it to do all the work. Prepping foods is very easy, too: just a little oil, some seasonings, and stick it in the cooking chamber. It's rare to find a recipe for an air-fried food longer than a few steps, so if you're someone who believes they could burn water, you'll love air-frying.

Versatility

You can make a lot of different foods in an air fryer. While the most common dishes include French fries and other snack foods, you can also make vegetables, kale chips, and meats like chicken wings and seafood. You can even make desserts like cake, cheesecake, and cookies, too. The air fryer is essentially a small oven, so if you can bake it, you can air-fry it.

Benefits of air fryers include fast preparation, the ability to make a wide variety of dishes, safe and easy use, and easy clean-up.

Safety

Air fryers are much safer than deep fryers, which can splatter scalding hot oil on anyone standing too close. In an air fryer, everything is contained. While the interior of an air fryer gets very hot in order to cook food, most models are built with cool-touch exteriors. They also all come with a cooling system that prevents too much pressure from building up inside the chamber. You can safely use the fryer with young kids and pets around.

Easy cleaning

Because air fryers use significantly less oil than deep fryers, cleaning them is much easier. They don't accumulate as much grime during the cooking process and you don't have to deal with a bath of used oil. On most models, you can remove parts like the cooking chamber and wash them in the dishwasher if you want. If you choose to handwash, it's a good idea to soak the chamber first if there's food or batter stuck inside it. Since air fryers use non-stick material, it's also easy to wipe the outside clean by hand.

Are air fryers healthy?

You might wonder why none of the benefits talked about health, so let's take a second to discuss that right now. The reality is that air-frying *is* healthier than deep-frying. It uses 80% less oil and reduces a food's calorie count by more than half compared to frying in an pan or deep-frying. However, air-frying is not guaranteed to help you lose weight or fit perfectly into a healthy lifestyle. It all depends on how often you use it and what you choose to make with it.

If you use your air fryer to prepare vegetables and you're eating more veggies this way than you would normally, you will experience health benefits. There are lots of great air-fried recipes for zucchini, kale, carrots, and more. You can even use the air fryer to make corn on the cob, asparagus, and roasted garlic. If you use it to make a lot of French fries and onion rings and you didn't eat that many before, you'll experience negative effects. Even switching to everyday air-fried "junk" foods after a diet heavy in regular fried foods probably won't make a huge difference for your health. Air-fried food is basically still fried food, so you want to limit how much you're eating. However, air-frying can definitely be part of a healthy lifestyle (while deep-frying can't really fit), and air-fried onion rings and French fries as a treat are a better alternative to deep-fried.

Downsides to air fryers

Air fryers are easy to use, produce tasty food, and reduce calories compared to deep-frying, but there are some concerns you should know about. Here are the most commonly-reported downsides that owners are talking about:

Food can burn easily

Since an air fryer gets so hot, food can turn from crispy and delicious to burned and gross very quickly. Even though they are safe, you never want to leave an air fryer by itself in case you chose the wrong cooking time and food starts to burn and smell. When looking at recipes, take a glance at the comments to make sure people who tried it aren't reporting burned results.

Burnt food is bad for you

If you burn a food, don't eat it. That black char contains a compound called acrylamide, which has been linked to cancer in some studies. Burnt food also just doesn't taste good. If the food isn't burned all over, you can scrape off the black part, but ideally, you want food that hasn't been charred at all.

Downsides of air fryers can include dry and burned food. Also, air-fried food isn't necessarily automatically "healthy;" it all depends on what you choose to make.

Food can get too dry

Without a lot of oil, food in an air fryer can dry out. Hot air sucks out moisture when it's crisping up the outside of food, but depending on the food, that can result in a too-dry product. If you're working with a food that doesn't naturally hold a lot of moisture, an extra spritz of oil would probably help.

II. WHAT TO CONSIDER WHEN BUYING AN AIR FRYER

There are six things everyone should think about when shopping for an air fryer: size, price, effectiveness, display, cleaning, and accessories. Since you're looking to make food for just you and one other person, you will be looking at every air fryer option through that lens. Let's break down your choices:

Size

Since you will only be cooking food for two people, you should look at the smaller air fryer options. How companies determine the size of their fryer can be a bit weird. Philips will say how many pounds of food a model can fit, so their 2.2-quart fryer holds 1.8 pounds of food. The 3.2-quart one cooks 2.6 pounds. Others will simply say quarts. The small ones range from 2.2-3.7 , while larger ones weigh 5-6 quarts. For two people, you probably want an air fryer between 3.0-5.8 quarts. Keep in mind that certain foods take up more space than others, so if you want to be able to cook a chicken dinner for two, you should make sure the air fryer is large enough.

Price

Air fryers range in price. They can be as cheap as under $100 and as expensive as close to $400. Size and features play a big role in the pricing, as well as brand. If you want a reliable fryer for two with basic features, you should be able to find several affordable options.

Effectiveness

Arguably the most important question to ask when looking at air fryers is how well it cooks food. You want one that cooks the food evenly and gets a beautiful crispy texture, so check out what people are saying about the one you're looking at. There are lots of blogs and articles where customers test foods like French fries, ribs, cupcakes, etc, and review how well the air fryer performed.

Display

What kind of display is "best" really depends on what you want - do you care if it's digital or not? Do you care about cooking programs? The digital air fryers with a bunch of presets will probably be on the higher end, price-wise. They do provide more precise cooking temperatures, which makes it easier to avoid overcooking the food. A well-made analog air fryer, however, beats a poorly-designed digital one any day, so don't assume digital is the only way to go.

Cleaning

You should also see what people are saying about cleaning the fryer you're considering. Does the air fryer have dishwasher-safe parts? Is the non-stick coating durable or does it flake off too soon? If you want to use your air fryer a lot, clean-up should be convenient.

> **When choosing an air fryer, consider factors like size, price, how well it air-fries, the display, how easy it is to clean, and what accessories are available. Good brands include Philips, Cuisinart, and T-Fal ActiFry.**

Accessories

The last thing you should know about air fryers is that they are very accessory-friendly. That means you can use extra equipment like a toast rack, pizza rack, or cake barrel to make a wider variety of food. Lots of companies make accessories you can buy separately, or if you have ramekins and other baking dishes that fit in your fryer, you can just use those. If it's oven-safe, it's air-fryer safe. Keep in mind that accessories like a cake barrel probably won't fit in an air fryer designed for feeding just two people. If you want to cook as many foods as possible, you should opt for a larger size.

Brands

According to Forbes, the best air fryers of 2018 came from these brands:

- Philips
- SimpleTaste
- T-Fal ActiFry
- Cuisinart
- Power Air Fryer
- Avalon Bay

You should also consider air fryers from GoWise, Black & Decker, and Gourmia.

III. HOW TO USE YOUR AIR FRYER

Once you've selected your air fryer and it's sitting on your countertop, how does it work? The process is pretty much the same no matter what brand you're using. There are just two steps: prep and frying.

Prep

Get out the food you're going to fry. Toss with no more than 2 tablespoons of oil. Since you're making food for just two people, it will most likely be around ½ tablespoon-1 tablespoon. If the recipe calls for a batter or flour, prepare that and dip your ingredients. If you're just reheating a frozen food, spritz with a light coat of oil instead of tossing it.

What oils are best for air-frying?

Air fryers get very hot, so you want what's known as a "high-smoke point oil." This means that the oil only begins to smoke at a very hot temperature. For air-frying, you want an oil with a 400-degree or higher smoke point. Coconut oil isn't good because it has a 350-degree smoke point. The most common oils for air fryers include plain ol' canola oil and light olive oil. Here are some other more interesting options if you want to shake things up:

Ghee - clarified butter, nuttier taste than regular butter

Sunflower - light oil without much flavor

Avocado - light oil with a slightly-fruity flavor

Grapeseed - fruity mild flavor

Walnut - very strong, nutty flavor

Peanut - strong nutty flavor

Sesame - strong flavor

Using an air fryer is easy. To prep food, apply a coating of high-smoke point oil like light olive oil, adjust the temperature and time since air fryers cook faster than ovens, and then cook! Shake the basket every 3-4 minutes to ensure even cooking if the fryer doesn't have automatic paddles.

Air-frying

When your air fryer is preheated and ready to go, add your food. If the food is battered, don't stack it; you want a single layer so everything cooks evenly. If it isn't battered and just lightly-sprayed with oil, stacking is okay. It just won't be as crispy. How long should you cook? And at what temperature? The general rule is is to reduce an oven temperature by 20-25% for an air fryer, and reduce cook time by 40-45% of the time in an oven. When you're first starting out, stick with the shorter time and cooler temp to make sure nothing overcooks. If the food ends up undercooked, you can always return it to the chamber for a few more minutes. There's no saving overcooked or burned food. If you're using a basket-style air fryer, you'll want to shake it every 3-4 minutes of cook time.

What kind of food can you make in an air fryer?

When buying a "specialized" kitchen application, you want to get your money's worth. What can the air fryer cook? The recipe section of this book will provide you with all kinds of meals and snacks, but let's just quickly go down a list of what you can make with an air fryer:

Breakfasts

- Hash browns
- Egg cups
- Burritos
- Frittatas

Snacks + sides

- Kale chips
- Apple chips
- Sweet potato fries
- French fries
- Onion rings
- Jalapeno poppers
- Vegetables
- Quick breads

You can make just about anything in air fryer, like hash browns, vegetable chips, chicken wings, seafood, donuts, and cakes.

Meals

- Tacos
- Taquitos
- Chicken wings
- Turkey wings
- Tofu
- Pork chops
- Fish fillets
- Shrimp
- Egg rolls
- Fish 'n chips
- Hot dogs
- Hamburgers

Sweets

- Donuts
- Cinnamon rolls
- Muffins
- Cakes
- Lava cakes
- Fruit crumbles
- Pop tarts

V. PROPER CARE AND MAINTENANCE

Air fryers are like any other kitchen appliance: they need to be used safely and taken care of. Keeping your fryer in the right place and checking for damage prevents accidents, while cleaning the fryer after cooking ensures that your fryer lasts as ong as possible and cooks delicious food every time.

Safety

When you get your air fryer, you want to set it up in the safest spot possible. It should rest on a level surface. Once you've had and used your fryer for a while, always make sure nothing has been damaged before turning it on. Look for frayed cords in particular, since starting an air fryer with a messed-up cord could result in electrocution or a fire. If you see a fray or tear, do not use the air fryer or try to tape it up. Get it repaired or replace it. While you're at it, look for any leftover food or dust on or in the fryer, and give it a quick wipedown.

Cleaning your fryer after use

Cleaning an air fryer after it's been used is very important. If you don't, it will smell and be a real pain to clean when you want to use it again. The first thing you should do is unplug the air fryer and wait for a complete cooldown. Once it's no longer warm, you can remove most of the parts, like the basket. Either wash by hand or run through the dishwasher. If there are still lingering smells after a wash, rinse out the chamber with a mixture of water, lemon juice, vinegar, and baking soda. If you're washing the fryer after each use, persistent smells shouldn't be a big problem.

For the outside of the fryer, all you need is a clean sponge and warm water. If there's food stuck on it, use a toothbrush to rub it off. Something too abrasive like steel wool is too intense and will scratch the surface.

When everything is clean, check that all the parts are dry before putting the fryer back together. When you're storing it, you want it to sit upright, like it does when it's in use. If you're not using it, keep it unplugged. It's just safer.

You should always clean your air fryer after using it. Be sure it's unplugged and completely cool before putting the removable parts in the dishwasher or washing by hand. You want to use a mild, natural degreasing soap like Method or Seventh Generation. Scrub with soft sponges and dry all the parts well.

What are the best soaps for degreasing?

The right soap can make a big difference. When you own an air fryer, oil and grease are part of life, so you want a product that can really cut through. There are four great choices that are also all-natural:

Better Life

The perfect dish soap for washing by hand, Better Life comes in a lemon-mint scent and contains aloe and Vitamin E, so your skin stays soft.

Method

Good Housekeeping reports that Method's dish soap works at removing grease and the pump design is convenient. You can get the soap in scents like Honeycrisp Apple.

Seventh Generation

A very effective degreasing soap, Seventh Generation uses botanical extracts, essential oils, and other natural ingredients. They offer an unscented version if you aren't a fan of fragrances.

This soap contains soap bark extract, which is very effective at removing grease, so a little goes a long way. Mrs. Meyer's has a lot of fragrance options and is made from 97% natural ingredients.

Air fryer troubleshooting

When you're new to air-frying, you might encounter some issues. What if your fryer starts smoking? What if the food is dry? The following fryer problems are the most commonly-reported:

Problem: Smoke or fumes

When you see white smoke rising out of your fryer, there are two possible reasons: the food is fatty or you used too much oil. Fatty foods tend to produce smoke when they're air-fried. You can stop the process and carefully soak up the oil on the pan or pour off the excess. You can also use a variety basket, splatter-proof lid, or snack cover for especially fat-rich foods. The other reason is too much oil. You want to carefully measure your oil because even an extra teaspoon can make a big difference.

White smoke doesn't actually hurt the air fryer; it's just steam. However, if the smoke is *black,* something is wrong. Talk to the manufacturer. If the smoke is blue, which is rare, you're dealing with an electrical problem and the heat is actually melting the plastic. Turn off and unplug the fryer immediately and don't use it again. It will most likely need to be replaced.

Air fryers can experience a few problems, such as smoke, a scratched or peeling interior, interrupted cooking, or dry food. Most issues can be solved easily or you should get the air fryer repaired or replaced.

Problem: Peeling, bubbles, or scratches on the inside lining

When you see damage like this on the inside of your fryer, it's most likely because it hasn't been cleaned properly. You've probably used something too harsh. Start cleaning a bit more carefully with soft sponges and gentle dish soaps. If you start seeing bits of the non-stick coating in your food, you probably need to replace the air fryer. High-quality fryer brands like Philips don't usually produce this kind of flaking if you take care of them.

Problem: Air fryer won't turn on or suddenly stops during cooking

If the air fryer won't start at all, check to make sure it's plugged in. It's the first rule for any electronic appliance. Check the outlet while you're at it, too; sometimes they get loose. If the air fryer suddenly stops in the middle of cooking, it could also be because of the outlet. Try a different plug to see if that fixes the problem.

If not, the problem probably lies with the air fryer. If the fryer is relatively new, contact the manufacturer and see if they'll replace it. You might also be able to get the air fryer repaired, though more often than not, getting a new one ends up costing less.

Problem: Dry, chewy, or soggy food

All three of these problems are caused by the same thing: not enough oil. When your food isn't coated by a layer of oil, the hot air from the fryer ends up baking everything. You won't get that crispy exterior. Always follow the air fryer recipe's recommendation for how much oil to use; don't use less to try to save a few calories. The food won't turn out the way you want.

VI. 15 TIPS FOR SUCCESS

You now know enough about air fryers to choose the best model for you and start cooking, but there are some additional tips that will ensure success every time you use your fryer. Here are the best 15 collected from various books, blogs, and brands:

Put the fryer in the right place

The perfect place for an air fryer is on a level counter about 4-5 inches from the wall. You don't want the fryer pressed right up against something or it won't be able to properly vent. That 4-5 inches also applies to the space *above* the fryer.

Always preheat the fryer

Before putting your oil-coated food into your air fryer, let the fryer preheat a little while. Putting food in while the fryer is cold could mess up the cooking time. Some recipes will say specifically not to preheat, but unless that's specifically stated, just preheat for 2-3 minutes.

Use a special spray bottle for oil

Spraying oil on your food is the best way to get an even coating. Avoid using aerosol cans (the oils often contain harsh chemicals) and instead get your own food-grade kitchen spray bottle. This way, you can fill it yourself and know the oil you're using is pure. Brushed stainless steel or glass are the most popular materials since they are durable and easy to clean.

Get a French fry cutter

Excited for homemade French fries? A French fry cutter is one of the best purchases you can make when you own an air fryer. These specialized cutters ensure uniform fries that turn out perfectly every time. A cutter is way faster than prepping fries by hand and will work for white and sweet potatoes.

Little actions like using a spray bottle for oil, adding water when cooking fatty foods, and making a foil sling for baking pans can make- air-frying even more convenient.

Get a mandolin slicer

Speaking of cutting, a mandoline slicer is a must-have if you want to increase your vegetable consumption. A mandolin slicer lets you cut veggies in a variety of thicknesses (usually three), so you end up with uniform cuts for veggie chips. It's also safer than trying to cut really thinly with a regular knife.

Bread properly

If your food calls for breading, always follow the same three-step process: flour coating, egg, and then crumbs. Sometimes the flour is replaced with cornstarch and the bread crumbs are cornflakes or something else that's been crushed, but egg should always be in the middle. Really roll the food around in the crumbs, so they stick. The fan in the air fryer can blow loose crumbs off otherwise.

Get parchment liners

You can get parchments liners specifically made for air fryers. They have a 9-inch diameter, so they fit in most air fryers, such as the 5.3-quart ones. You could cut out your own, but that takes a lot of time. The benefit of using a liner is that clean-up is much easier. Keep in mind that most liners will be okay at a max of 450-degrees for 20 minutes.

If you're making something fatty, add water

We talked about how air-frying fatty foods can cause white smoke. One way to prevent this is to pour a little water into the cooking drawer below the food. This prevents any fat from dripping down directly on the hot surface and producing smoke.

Flip foods at the halfway mark

If you want foods to be perfectly-evenly cooked, flip them halfway through the cooking time like you would in an oven. This step is often written into recipes, but it won't be included in all of them, so just keep it in your head to do it. It can only make food better.

Spray with a bit more oil at the halfway point for extra crisp

If you are really into a good crisp on your food, spray what you're making with a little oil halfway through cooking. A lot of people find air-frying doesn't get quite as crispy as they're used to, so spraying on some extra oil partway through might help.

After cooking meat, use the leftover juice for a sauce

While marinated meat cooks in the air fryer, delicious juice will drip down into the drawer. When cook time is over, carefully remove the drawer and pour the juice into a saucepan to make a gravy or sauce. Reduce over medium heat for a rich taste. For thickness, add a bit of a cornstarch/water mixture. If you want to try this out, skip adding water into the drawer and expect to see some white smoke if the meat is fatty. As mentioned earlier, this white smoke doesn't hurt your air fryer.

To keep food moist, wrap in tin foil

It's safe to wrap food in foil when it's being air-fried. You just have to make sure the wrapped items are about ¾ of an inch away from the air fryer's edge. The food will cook evenly this way. You should also poke holes in the top of the foil, so excess moisture can escape and the food won't steam-cook. What about a crispy exterior? Simply remove the foil during the last few minutes of cooking. Foods that are really good when foil-wrapped include brownies, muffins, prawns, and squash.

Make a foil sling for easy accessory removal

Getting cake pans and other baking dishes out of the air fryer can be tricky since most of them will be a snug fit. For easy removal, make a foil sling. Fold out a piece that's about 2-inches wide and 24-inches long. Put the foil in the air fryer so the two ends are outside. The dish will go on top of the foil in the fryer with the two ends tucked on top of that, so you can close the drawer. When cook time is up, you simply unfold the ends and lift.

Hold light foods down with toothpicks

With the fan in the fryer blowing away, light foods sometimes get rearranged during the cooking process. For example, if you're air-frying a panini, the top slice of bread might move around. To prevent this from happening, use a toothpick to keep everything in place.

Reheat food with the air fryer

You can use the air fryer even when food has already been fully-cooked. Leftovers get dried out when you microwave them and the oven can take too long. Why not use the air fryer? That way, the food won't be bone-dry or too soggy. A good temperature for just about any reheated food is 350-degrees. If you're reheating meat, just make sure the internal temp gets up to the recommended number.

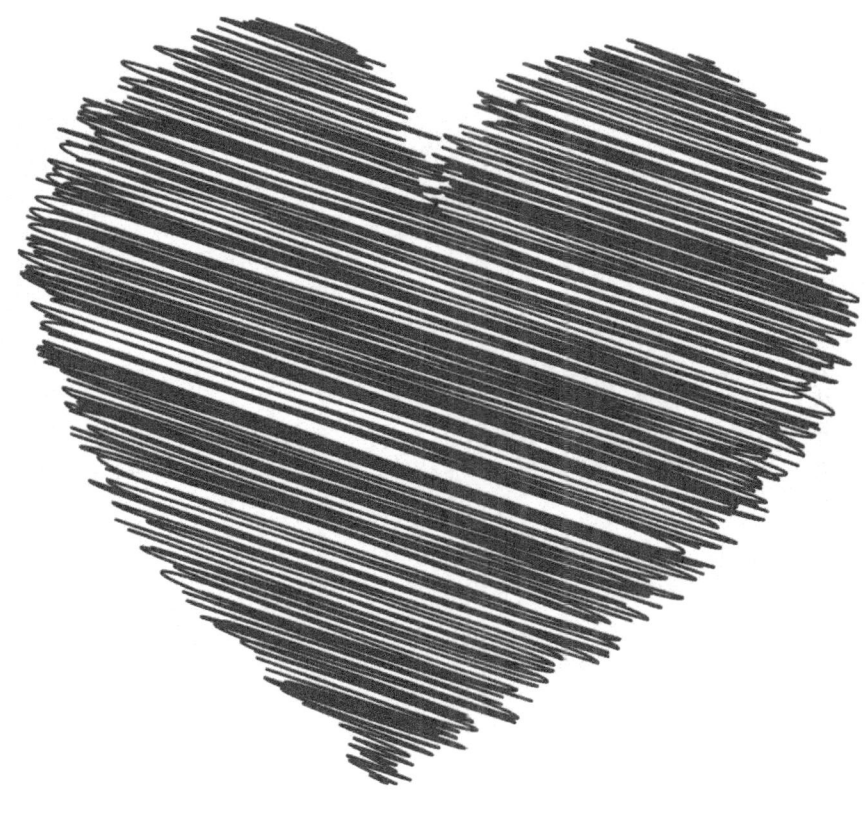

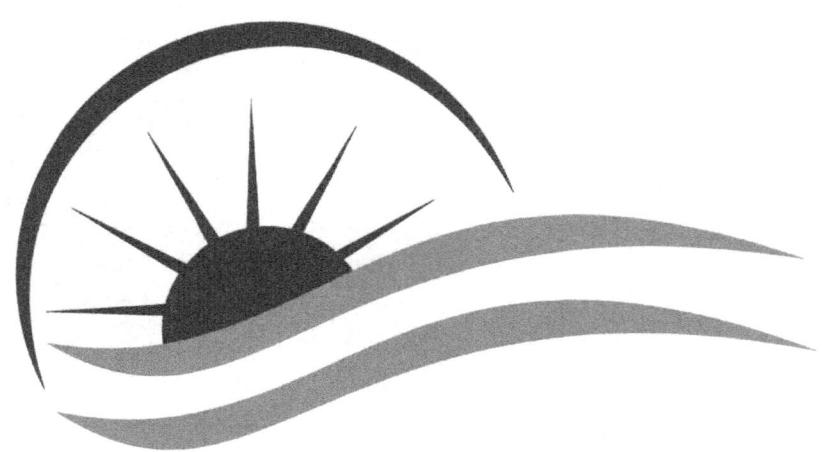

BREAKFAST RECIPES

Contents

CHEESE SANDWICH

Total Time: 15 minutes

Serves: 2

Ingredients:
- 4 cheddar cheese slices
- 4 tsp butter
- 4 bread slices

Directions:
- Place 2 cheese slices between the 2 bread slices and spread the butter outside of both the bread slices.
- Assemble remaining sandwich using the same step.
- Place sandwich in air fryer basket and cook at 187 C/ 370 F for 8 minutes. Turn halfway through.
- Serve and enjoy.

Nutritional Value (Amount per Serving):
- Calories 341
- Fat 26.8 g
- Carbohydrates 9.8 g
- Sugar 1.1 g
- Protein 15.4 g
- Cholesterol 79 mg

BREAKFAST FRITTATA

Total Time: 25 minutes

Serves: 2

Ingredients:

- 1 cup egg whites
- 2 tbsp chives, chopped
- 1/4 cup mushrooms, sliced
- 1/4 cup tomato, sliced
- 2 tbsp milk
- Pepper
- Salt

Directions:

- Preheat the air fryer at 160 C/ 320 F.
- In a bowl, whisk together all ingredients.
- Spray frying pan with cooking spray. (frying pan which you get with your air fryer)
- Transfer frittata mixture to the pan and place in air fryer basket.
- Bake frittata in preheated air fryer for 15 minutes.
- Serve and enjoy.

Nutritional Value (Amount per Serving):

- Calories 78
- Fat 0.6 g
- Carbohydrates 3 g
- Sugar 2.4 g
- Protein 14.3 g
- Cholesterol 1 mg

FRENCH TOAST

Total Time: 15 minutes

Serves: 2

Ingredients:

- 4 bread slices
- 1 tbsp cinnamon
- 1 tsp vanilla
- 2/3 cup milk
- 2 eggs

Directions:

- In a small bowl, mix together eggs, vanilla, cinnamon, and milk until well combined.
- Dip each bread slices into the egg mixture and shake excess of the egg mixture. Place bread slice in a pan.
- Place pan in air fryer and cook at 160 C/ 320 F for 3 minutes then turn to other side and cook for 3 minutes more.
- Serve and enjoy.

Nutritional Value (Amount per Serving):

- Calories 166
- Fat 6.7 g
- Carbohydrates 16.5 g
- Sugar 5.1 g
- Protein 9.7 g
- Cholesterol 170 mg

SIMPLE BROCCOLI FRITTATA

Total Time: 30 minutes

Serves: 2

Ingredients:

- 3 eggs
- 2 tbsp parmesan cheese, grated
- 2 tbsp milk
- 1/2 cup bell pepper, chopped
- 1/2 cup broccoli florets
- Pepper
- Salt

Directions:

- Spray baking dish with cooking spray.
- Place bell peppers and broccoli in the prepared baking dish.
- Cook broccoli and bell pepper at 176 C/ 350 F for 7 minutes.
- In a bowl, whisk together eggs, milk, and seasoning.
- Once veggies are cooked then add egg mixture and sprinkle grated cheese on top.
- Cook in air fryer for 10 minutes more.
- Serve and enjoy.

Nutritional Value (Amount per Serving):

- Calories 157
- Fat 9.3 g
- Carbohydrates 5.1 g
- Sugar 3.1 g
- Protein 12.8 g
- Cholesterol 254 mg

SIMPLE BREAKFAST SOUFFLÉ

Total Time: 15 minutes

Serves: 2

Ingredients:
- 2 eggs
- 1 tbsp parsley, chopped
- 1/4 tsp red chili pepper
- 2 tbsp cream
- Pepper
- Salt

Directions:
- Spray four ramekins with cooking spray and set aside.
- Whisk eggs in a bowl and stir in red chili pepper, parsley, cream, pepper, and salt.
- Pour egg mixture into the prepared ramekins.
- Place ramekins into the air fryer basket and bake at 200 C/ 392 F for 8 minutes.
- Serve and enjoy.

Nutritional Value (Amount per Serving):
- Calories 72
- Fat 5.1 g
- Carbohydrates 0.9 g
- Sugar 0.6 g
- Protein 5.7 g
- Cholesterol 166 mg

DELICIOUS BREAKFAST FRITTATA

Total Time: 25 minutes

Serves: 2

Ingredients:

- 2 large eggs
- 1 tbsp butter, melted
- 2 tbsp cheddar cheese
- 1 tbsp bell peppers, chopped
- 1 tbsp spring onions, chopped
- 1 breakfast sausage patty, chopped
- Pepper
- Salt

Directions:

- Spray 4" mini pan with cooking spray and set aside.
- Add chopped sausage patty in prepared dish and air fry at 176 C/ 350 F for 5 minutes.
- Meanwhile, in a bowl whisk together eggs, pepper, and salt.
- Add bell peppers, spring onions and mix well.
- Once sausages are done then add egg mixture and mix well.
- Sprinkle with cheese and air fry at 176 C/ 350 F for 5 minutes.
- Serve hot and enjoy.

Nutritional Value (Amount per Serving):

- Calories 206
- Fat 14.7 g
- Carbohydrates 6.7 g
- Sugar 4 g
- Protein 12.8 g
- Cholesterol 221 mg

TOAST SOLDIERS

Total Time: 15 minutes

Serves: 2

Ingredients:

- 4 bread slices
- 1 tsp cinnamon
- 1 tbsp honey
- 1/4 cup brown sugar
- 1/4 cup milk
- 2 eggs
- 1/8 tsp nutmeg

Directions:

- Cut bread slices into soldiers. Cut each bread slice in four soldiers.
- In a bowl, mix together remaining ingredients until well combined.
- Coat each soldier with bowl mixture and place in air fryer basket.
- Cook at 160 C/320 F for 10 minutes. Turn halfway through.
- Serve with fresh berries and enjoy.

Nutritional Value (Amount per Serving):

- Calories 230
- Fat 5.6 g
- Carbohydrates 38.4 g
- Sugar 28.8 g
- Protein 8 g
- Cholesterol 166 mg

SCRAMBLED EGGS

Total Time: 15 minutes

Serves: 2

Ingredients:

- 4 eggs
- 2 bread slices
- Pepper
- Salt

Directions:

- Warm bread slices at 200 C/ 400 F for 3 minutes.
- Crack eggs into the pan. This fits into the air fryer.
- Season eggs with pepper and salt. Stir well.
- Place pan in air fryer and cook at 180 C/ 360 F for 2 minutes. Stir quickly and cook for 4 minutes more.
- Stir well and transfer the scrambled eggs over the toasted bread slices.
- Serve warm and enjoy.

Nutritional Value (Amount per Serving):

- Calories 150
- Fat 9.1 g
- Carbohydrates 5.3 g
- Sugar 1.1 g
- Protein 11.8 g
- Cholesterol 327 mg

HEALTHY GRANOLA BARS

Total Time: 20 minutes

Serves: 2

Ingredients:

- 1 1/2 cups oats
- 1/2 tsp cinnamon
- 1/2 tsp vanilla
- 1/2 tbsp olive oil
- 1/2 apple, peeled and cooked
- 1 1/2 tbsp honey
- 1/2 oz brown sugar
- 1 oz butter, melted
- 3 tbsp raisins

Directions:

- Add oats to the blender and blend until smooth. Add remaining dry ingredients and mix well.
- In an air fryer, baking pan add all wet ingredients and stir well.
- Add oats mixture to the baking pan and mix well.
- Add raisins and press down the mixture in baking pan. Make sure mixture is in level.
- Cook at 160 C/ 320 F for 10 minutes. Cook for another 5 minutes at 180 C/ 360 F.
- Place in the refrigerator for 5 minutes to stiff the bar mixture.
- Cut into bars and serve.

Nutritional Value (Amount per Serving):

- Calories 513
- Fat 19.2 g
- Carbohydrates 80.5 g
- Sugar 34.4 g
- Protein 8.8 g
- Cholesterol 30 mg

SIMPLE EGG CUPS

Total Time: 15 minutes

Serves: 2

Ingredients:
- 1/4 cup egg beaters
- 4 tsp jack cheese, shredded
- 4 tbsp spinach, chopped
- 4 tbsp sausage, cooked and crumbled
- Pepper
- Salt

Directions:
- In a mixing bowl, whisk together all ingredients until well combined.
- Pour batter into the muffin cups and place in air fryer basket.
- Bake at 165 C/ 330 F for 10 minutes.
- Allow to cool completely then serve.

Nutritional Value (Amount per Serving):
- Calories 89
- Fat 6.3 g
- Carbohydrates 1 g
- Sugar 0.2 g
- Protein 7 g
- Cholesterol 14 mg

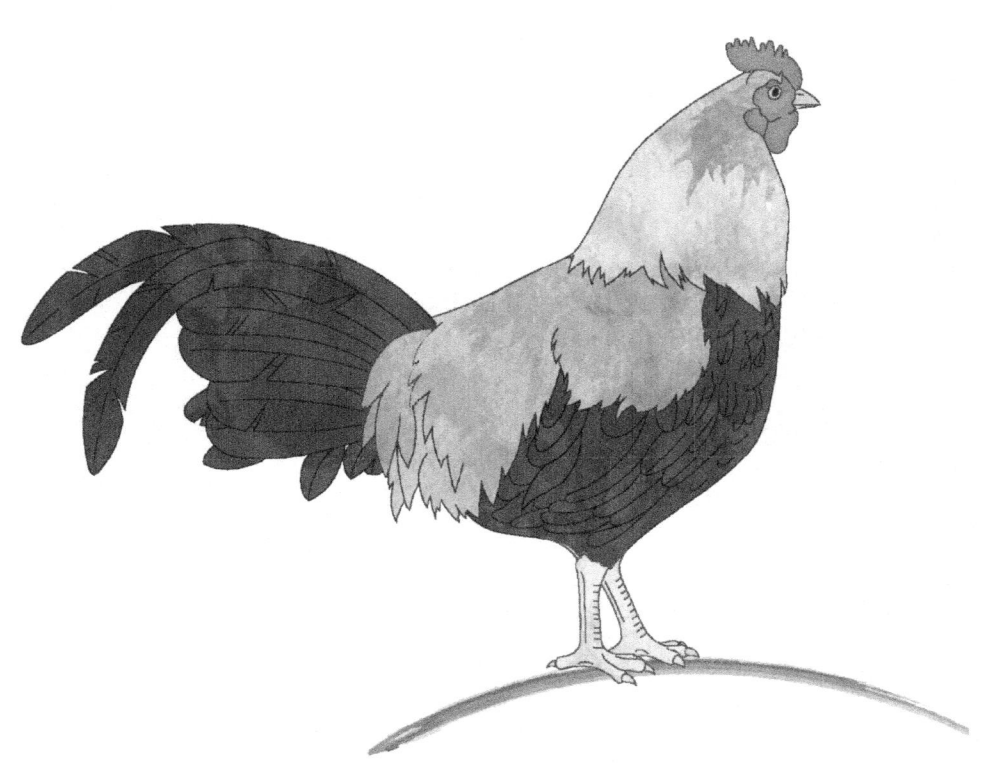

CHICKEN RECIPES

Contents

SPICY CHICKEN NUGGETS

Total Time: 30 minutes

Serves: 2

Ingredients:
- 1/2 lb chicken, boneless
- 1/2 cup breadcrumbs
- 1 1/2 tbsp fresh coriander, chopped
- 1 tbsp olive oil
- 1 tbsp lemon juice
- 1/2 tbsp ginger garlic paste
- 1 tsp garam masala
- 1 tsp cumin powder
- 1/2 tsp chili powder
- 1/2 tsp red chili flakes
- Salt

Directions:
- Preheat the air fryer to 356 F/ 180 C.
- In a mixing bowl, add all ingredients except breadcrumbs and mix well.
- Marinate chicken for 30 minutes.
- Coat marinated chicken with breadcrumbs and place in air fryer basket and cook for 15-20 minutes.
- Serve hot and enjoy.

Nutritional Value (Amount per Serving):
- Calories 346
- Fat 12.3 g
- Carbohydrates 20.4 g
- Sugar 1.9 g
- Protein 36.8 g
- Cholesterol 87 mg

BUFFALO CHICKEN WINGS

Total Time: 30 minutes

Serves: 2

Ingredients:

- 1/4 cup hot sauce
- 1/2 lb chicken wings

Directions:

- Preheat the air fryer at 204 C/ 400 F for 4-5 minutes.
- Place chicken wings in the air fryer basket and air fry for 12 minutes.
- Turn wings to other side and air fry for 10-12 minutes more.
- Transfer wings to the bowl. Add hot sauce and mix well.
- Serve and enjoy.

Nutritional Value (Amount per Serving):

- Calories 219
- Fat 8.5 g
- Carbohydrates 0.5 g
- Sugar 0.4 g
- Protein 33 g
- Cholesterol 101 mg

SPICY CHICKEN WINGS

Total Time: 25 minutes

Serves: 2

Ingredients:

- 1 lb chicken wings
- 1 1/2 tbsp butter, melted
- 2 tbsp hot sauce
- Salt
- For finishing sauce:
- 2 tbsp hot sauce
- 1 1/2 tbsp butter, melted

Directions

- Add chicken wings, hot sauce, butter, and salt in a mixing bowl and mix until well coated.
- Place marinated chicken wings in the refrigerator for 2 hours.
- Preheat the air fryer to 204 C/ 400 F.
- Add marinated chicken wings into the air fryer basket and air fry for 12 minutes.
- Meanwhile, in a large bowl combine together hot sauce and melted butter.
- Remove chicken wings from air fryer and place in hot sauce mixture. Toss well to coat.
- Serve and enjoy.

Nutritional Value (Amount per Serving):

- Calories 585
- Fat 34.1 g
- Carbohydrates 0.3 g
- Sugar 0.2 g
- Protein 65.9 g
- Cholesterol 248 mg

CRISP CHICKEN TENDERS

Total Time: 25 minutes

Serves: 2

Ingredients:

- 1 egg
- 4 piece chicken tenders
- 1/2 tsp Italian herbs
- 1/4 cup parmesan cheese, grated
- 1/2 cup breadcrumbs
- 1/2 tsp garlic powder
- 1 1/2 tbsp butter, melted

Directions

- In a bowl, combine together egg, Italian herbs, garlic powder, and butter.
- Add chicken tenders in egg mixture and coat well.
- In a shallow dish, combine together parmesan cheese and breadcrumbs.
- Coat chicken with cheese and breadcrumbs mixture and set aside for 5 minutes.
- Spray air fryer basket with cooking spray.
- Preheat the air fryer to 200 C/ 392 F for 3 minutes.
- Place chicken tenders in air fryer basket and air fry for 6 minutes.
- Serve hot and enjoy.

Nutritional Value (Amount per Serving):

- Calories 626
- Fat 34.3 g
- Carbohydrates 43.7 g
- Sugar 2 g
- Protein 37.8 g
- Cholesterol 167 mg

TASTY CHICKEN TIKKA

Total Time: 30 minutes

Serves: 2

Ingredients:

- 1/2 lb boneless chicken, cut into pieces
- 1/2 cup yogurt
- 1 bell peppers, cut into chunks
- 1/2 cup cherry tomatoes
- 1/2 tsp turmeric powder
- 1 tbsp coriander powder
- 1 tbsp cumin powder
- 1/2 tbsp ginger garlic paste
- 1 tbsp red chili powder
- 1 tsp olive oil
- Salt

Directions

- Add all ingredients into the large bowl and place in refrigerator for 2 hours.
- Threading marinated chicken, pepper, and tomatoes alternately on skewers.
- Preheat the air fryer to 200 C/ 392 F for 5 minutes.
- Line air fryer basket with foil and place chicken skewers on foil.
- Grill for 15 minutes. Turn skewers once.
- Serve and enjoy.

Nutritional Value (Amount per Serving):

- Calories 331
- Fat 13.1 g
- Carbohydrates 14.3 g
- Sugar 8.9 g
- Protein 38.3 g
- Cholesterol 107 mg

CHICKEN SKEWER

Total Time: 30 minutes

Serves: 2

Ingredients:

- 1/2 lb chicken tenders
- 1/2 tsp ginger, minced
- 3/4 tbsp soy sauce
- 2 garlic cloves, minced
- 1/2 tbsp sesame oil
- 50 ml pineapple juice
- 1/4 tsp pepper

Directions

- Preheat the air fryer to 198 C/390 F.
- In a bowl, combine together all ingredients except chicken.
- Skewer chicken tenders then place in a bowl and marinate for 2 hours.
- Air fry at 198 C/ 390 F for 18 minutes.
- Serve and enjoy.

Nutritional Value (Amount per Serving):

- Calories 269
- Fat 11.9 g
- Carbohydrates 5.4 g
- Sugar 2.8 g
- Protein 33.6 g
- Cholesterol 101 mg

CHICKEN NUGGETS

Total Time: 20 minutes

Serves: 2

Ingredients:

- 8 oz chicken breasts, cut into 1 " pieces
- 1 tbsp parmesan cheese
- 4 tbsp Italian seasoned breadcrumbs
- 1 tsp olive oil
- Pepper
- Salt

Directions:

- Preheat the air fryer to 204 C/ 400 F for 5 minutes.
- Take two bowls. Add olive oil in the first bowl. Add bread crumbs and cheese in seconds bowl.
- Season chicken with pepper and salt.
- Place chicken into the oiled bowl and mix well.
- Transfer chicken to the breadcrumbs mixture and coat well.
- Place coated chicken pieces into the air fryer basket. Spray chicken on top using cooking spray.
- Air fry at 204 C/ 400 F for 8 minutes. Turn halfway through.
- Serve and enjoy.

Nutritional Value (Amount per Serving):

- Calories 288
- Fat 11.8 g
- Carbohydrates 8.1 g
- Sugar 0.8 g
- Protein 35.3 g
- Cholesterol 103 mg

PARMESAN CHICKEN

Total Time: 20 minutes

Serves: 2

Ingredients:

- 8 oz chicken breast, cut in half
- 1/4 cup marinara
- 3 tbsp mozzarella cheese
- 1/2 tbsp olive oil
- 1 tbsp parmesan cheese
- 3 tbsp bread crumbs

Directions:

- Preheat the air fryer at 182 C/ 360 F for 5 minutes.
- Spray air fryer basket with cooking spray.
- Take two bowls, add parmesan cheese and breadcrumbs in the first bowl.
- Add olive oil in the second bowl.
- Brush chicken with olive oil and dip in breadcrumb mixture.
- Place coated chicken pieces into the air fryer basket and spray the top with cooking spray.
- Air fry for 6 minutes. Turn and top with marinara sauce and shredded mozzarella cheese.
- Air fry for 3 minutes more or until cheese is melted.
- Serve and enjoy.

Nutritional Value (Amount per Serving):

- Calories 349
- Fat 16.1 g
- Carbohydrates 11 g
- Sugar 0.6 g
- Protein 38.9 g
- Cholesterol 98 mg

HONEY CHICKEN WINGS

Total Time: 40 minutes

Serves: 2

Ingredients:

- 1 lb chicken wings
- 1/2 lime juice
- 1 tbsp butter
- 1 1/2 tbsp soy sauce
- 2 tbsp sriracha sauce
- 1/4 cup honey

Directions:

- Preheat the air fryer at 182 C/ 360 F.
- Add a chicken wing to the air fryer basket and cook for 30 minutes. Turn after every 7 minutes.
- Meanwhile, add remaining ingredients into the saucepan and bring to boil for 3 minutes.
- Once wings are cooked then toss them in a sauce until well coated.
- Serve and enjoy.

Nutritional Value (Amount per Serving):

- Calories 720
- Fat 32.6 g
- Carbohydrates 37.8 g
- Sugar 36.2 g
- Protein 66.6 g
- Cholesterol 227 mg

PARMESAN GARLIC CHICKEN WINGS

Total Time: 30 minutes

Serves: 2

Ingredients:

- 8 chicken wings, wash and pat dry
- 1/2 tsp garlic powder
- 1 tbsp soy sauce
- 2 tbsp parmesan cheese, grated
- 1/4 cup flour
- 2 tbsp buttermilk

Directions:

- Spray air fryer basket with cooking spray.
- Drizzle chicken wings with soy sauce and season with seasoning.
- Place chicken wings into the zip-lock bag and place in refrigerator for overnight.
- Add flour and parmesan in another zip-lock bag.
- Add buttermilk into the bowl. Add marinated chicken wings to the buttermilk and coat well.
- Now transfer chicken wings to the flour and parmesan mixture bag and shake well to coat.
- Place coated chicken wings to the air fryer basket and air fry at 204 C/ 400 F for 20 minutes. Shake air fryer basket after every 5 minutes.
- Serve and enjoy.

Nutritional Value (Amount per Serving):

- Calories 209
- Fat 9.6 g
- Carbohydrates 17.5 g
- Sugar 1.1 g
- Protein 13.6 g
- Cholesterol 35 mg

DELICIOUS CHICKEN JALFREZI

Total Time: 25 minutes

Serves: 2

Ingredients:

- 1/2 lb chicken thighs, skinless, boneless, and cut into 2" pieces
- 1/4 tsp cayenne
- 1/2 tsp garam masala
- 1/2 tsp turmeric
- 1 tbsp olive oil
- 1 cup bell pepper, chopped
- 1/2 cup onion, chopped
- 1/2 tsp salt
- For sauce:
- 1 tbsp tomato sauce
- 1/4 tsp cayenne
- 1/4 tsp salt
- 1/2 tsp garam masala
- 1/2 tbsp water

Directions:

- In a mixing bowl, mix together chicken, cayenne, garam masala, turmeric, olive oil, peppers, and onions.
- Place chicken mixture into the air fryer basket.
- Air fry at 182 C/ 360 F for 15 minutes. Toss halfway through.
- Meanwhile, for the sauce: In a microwave safe bowl, mix together all sauce ingredients and microwave for 1 minute.
- Remove from microwave and stir well and microwave for 1 minute more. Set aside.
- Once the chicken is cooked, transfer chicken and vegetable to the bowl.
- Pour prepared sauce over chicken and toss well to coat.
- Serve and enjoy.

Nutritional Value (Amount per Serving):

- Calories 311
- Fat 15.7 g
- Carbohydrates 8.2 g
- Sugar 4.6 g
- Protein 34 g
- Cholesterol 101 mg

FLAVORS HERB CHICKEN ROAST

Total Time: 35 minutes

Serves: 2

Ingredients:

- 10 oz chicken breast halves
- 1/4 tsp black pepper
- 1/4 tsp garlic powder
- 1/4 tsp dried rosemary
- 1/4 tsp dried thyme
- 1/4 tsp paprika
- 1 tbsp butter
- 1/4 tsp salt

Directions:

- In a small bowl, combine together butter, black pepper, garlic powder, rosemary, thyme, paprika, and salt.
- Rub butter mixture on both the chicken halves and place into the air fryer basket.
- Air fry at 190 C/ 375 F for 25 minutes.
- Serve and enjoy.

Nutritional Value (Amount per Serving):

- Calories 324
- Fat 16.3 g
- Carbohydrates 0.7 g
- Sugar 0.1 g
- Protein 41.2 g
- Cholesterol 141 mg

PESTO CHICKEN LEGS

Total Time: 30 minutes

Serves: 2

Ingredients:

- 4 chicken drumsticks
- 2 tbsp lemon juice
- 2 tbsp olive oil
- 1 tbsp ginger, slices
- 8 garlic cloves
- 1/2 jalapeno pepper
- 1/2 cup cilantro
- 1 tsp salt

Directions:

- Add all the ingredients except chicken into the blender and blend until smooth.
- Pour blended mixture into the large bowl.
- Add chicken into the bowl and stir well to coat. Place marinated chicken in refrigerator for 2 hours.
- Spray air fryer basket with cooking spray.
- Place marinated chicken to the air fryer basket and air fry at 198 C/390 F for 20 minutes. Turn halfway through.
- Serve and enjoy.

Nutritional Value (Amount per Serving):

- Calories 308
- Fat 19.6 g
- Carbohydrates 6.6 g
- Sugar 0.7 g
- Protein 26.6 g
- Cholesterol 81 mg

HEALTHY FENNEL CHICKEN

Total Time: 25 minutes

Serves: 2

Ingredients:

- 1/2 lb chicken thighs, skinless, boneless, and cut each thigh into 3 pieces
- 14 tsp cayenne pepper
- 1/2 tsp turmeric
- 1/2 tsp garam masala
- 1/2 tsp ground fennel seeds
- 1/2 tsp paprika
- 1 tsp garlic, minced
- 1 tsp ginger, minced
- 1/2 tbsp olive oil
- 1/2 onion, sliced
- 1/2 tsp salt

Directions:

- In a large mixing bowl, mix together all ingredients and allow the chicken to marinate for overnight.
- Place marinated chicken and veggies into the air fryer basket.
- Spray chicken mixture with cooking spray.
- Air fry at 182 C/ 360 F for 15 minutes. Turn halfway through.
- Serve and enjoy.

Nutritional Value (Amount per Serving):

- Calories 308
- Fat 19.6 g
- Carbohydrates 6.6 g
- Sugar 0.7 g
- Protein 26.6 g
- Cholesterol 81 mg

QUICK AND PERFECT CHICKEN BREAST

Total Time: 13 minutes

Serves: 2

Ingredients:
- 2 chicken breast
- 2 tsp olive oil
- Pepper
- Salt

Directions:
- Remove air fryer basket and replace it with air fryer grill pan.
- Place chicken breast to the grill pan.
- Season chicken with pepper and salt. Drizzle with olive oil.
- Air fry chicken at 175 C/ 375 F for 12 minutes.
- Serve and enjoy.

Nutritional Value (Amount per Serving):
- Calories 168
- Fat 7.5 g
- Carbohydrates 0 g
- Sugar 0 g
- Protein 23.8 g
- Cholesterol 72 mg

SHREDDED CHICKEN

Total Time: 20 minutes

Serves: 2

Ingredients:

- 2 large chicken breasts
- 1 tsp garlic puree
- 1 tsp mustard
- 1 tsp honey
- Pepper
- Salt

Directions:

- Add all ingredients to the bowl and mix well.
- Transfer chicken into the air fryer basket.
- Air fry chicken at 180 C/ 360 F for 15 minutes.
- Remove chicken from air fryer and shred using a fork.
- Serve and enjoy.

Nutritional Value (Amount per Serving):

- Calories 298
- Fat 11.3 g
- Carbohydrates 3.9 g
- Sugar 3 g
- Protein 42.8 g
- Cholesterol 130 mg

STICKY CHICKEN DRUMSTICKS

Total Time: 15 minutes

Serves: 2

Ingredients:

- 2 chicken drumsticks
- 1/2 tsp garlic paste
- 1/2 tsp mustard
- 1 tsp honey
- 1/2 tbsp olive oil
- Pepper
- Salt

Directions:

- Add all ingredients to the large bowl and mix well.
- Add chicken into the air fryer basket.
- Air fry at 175 C/ 347 F for 13 minutes.
- Serve and enjoy.

Nutritional Value (Amount per Serving):

- Calories 123
- Fat 6.4 g
- Carbohydrates 3.4 g
- Sugar 2.9 g
- Protein 12.9 g
- Cholesterol 40 mg

SWEET AND SPICY CHICKEN WINGS

Total Time: 40 minutes

Serves: 2

Ingredients:

- 1 lb chicken wings
- 1/2 tsp pepper
- 1/2 tsp salt
- For sauce:
- 1 tsp sugar
- 1/2 tbsp garlic, minced
- 1.2 tbsp ginger, minced
- 1/2 tbsp sesame oil
- 1/2 tsp honey
- 1/2 tbsp mayonnaise
- 1 tbsp gochujang (red chili paste)

Directions:

- Preheat the air fryer to 204 C/ 400 F.
- Add chicken wings into the air fryer basket and seasor with pepper and salt.
- Air fry chicken for 20 minutes.
- Meanwhile, in a bowl mix together all sauce ingredients.
- Add chicken wings to the sauce bowl and mix well.
- Transfer chicken wings to the air fryer basket again and air fry for 5 minutes.
- Serve and enjoy.

Nutritional Value (Amount per Serving):

- Calories 504
- Fat 21.7 g
- Carbohydrates 7.6 g
- Sugar 3.8 g
- Protein 66.1 g
- Cholesterol 203 mg

CLASSIC CHICKEN BURGERS

Total Time: 25 minutes

Serves: 2

Ingredients:

- 2 cups chicken minced
- 1/2 tbsp oregano
- 1 oz mozzarella cheese
- 1.75 oz breadcrumbs
- Pepper
- Salt

Directions:

- Add 3/4 bread crumbs, minced chicken, cheese, oregano, pepper, and salt into the mixing bowl and mix well to combine.
- Make small patties from chicken mixture and roll in remaining breadcrumbs.
- Place chicken burgers into the air fryer basket and cook at 180 C/ 360 F for 18 minutes
- Serve and enjoy.

Nutritional Value (Amount per Serving):

- Calories 353
- Fat 8.2 g
- Carbohydrates 19.1 g
- Sugar 1.6 g
- Protein 48 g
- Cholesterol 115 mg

BBQ CHICKEN WINGS

Total Time: 35 minutes

Serves: 2

Ingredients:

- 6 chicken wings
- 1/4 cup honey
- 1/4 cup BBQ sauce
- 1/4 cup flour
- 1/2 tsp pepper
- 1/2 tsp salt

Directions:

- Preheat the air fryer to 176 C/ 350 F.
- Add chicken wings, flour, pepper, and salt into the bowl and coat well.
- Place chicken wings into the air fryer basket and cook for 12 minutes. Turn chicken wings and cook for 12 minutes more.
- Meanwhile, in a bowl, mix together BBQ sauce and honey.
- Once chicken wings are cooked remove from air fryer and place into the sauce bowl.
- Coat well and serve.

Nutritional Value (Amount per Serving):

- Calories 530
- Fat 20.1 g
- Carbohydrates 58.5 g
- Sugar 43 g
- Protein 29.2 g
- Cholesterol 86 mg

SOUTHWEST CHICKEN

Total Time: 40 minutes

Serves: 2

Ingredients:

- 1/2 lb chicken breasts, skinless and boneless
- 1/8 tsp garlic powder
- 1/8 tsp onion powder
- 1/4 tsp cumin
- 1/4 tsp chili powder
- 1/2 tbsp olive oil
- 1 tbsp lime juice
- 1/8 tsp salt

Directions:

- Add all ingredients into the zip-lock bag and shake well and place in the fridge for 1 hour.
- Add a marinated chicken wing to the air fryer basket.
- Air fryer at 204 C/ 400 F for 25 minutes. Turn halfway through.
- Serve and enjoy.

Nutritional Value (Amount per Serving):

- Calories 249
- Fat 12 g
- Carbohydrates 0.6 g
- Sugar 0.1 g
- Protein 33 g
- Cholesterol 101 mg

HOT AND SPICY CHICKEN WINGS

Total Time: 30 minutes

Serves: 2

Ingredients:
- 6 chicken wings
- 1 tsp hot paprika
- 1 tbsp olive oil
- Pepper
- Salt

Directions:
- Preheat the air fryer to 200 C/ 392 F.
- In a bowl, mix together chicken, paprika, olive oil, pepper, and salt.
- Place marinated chicken into the fridge for 1 hour.
- Add marinated chicken into the air fryer basket and air fry for 12 minutes.
- Shake chicken wings well and cook for 8 minutes more.
- Serve hot and enjoy.

Nutritional Value (Amount per Serving):
- Calories 539
- Fat 39.2 g
- Carbohydrates 16.7 g
- Sugar 0.1 g
- Protein 29.4 g
- Cholesterol 116 mg

GARLIC CHEESE CHICKEN WINGS

Total Time: 35 minutes

Serves: 2

Ingredients:

- 1 lb chicken wings
- 1/8 tsp paprika
- 1/2 tsp oregano
- 1/2 tsp rosemary
- 1 garlic clove, minced
- 2 tbsp butter
- 2 tbsp parmesan cheese, grated
- 1/4 tsp salt

Directions:

- Preheat the air fryer to 200 C/ 392 F.
- Add chicken wings into the air fryer basket and cook for 24 minutes. Shake basket during the cooking process.
- Meanwhile, for sauce melt butter in a pan over medium heat.
- Add garlic and sauté for 30 seconds.
- Mix together herb and spices and add them into the pan.
- Once chicken wings are cooked then pour sauce over them.
- Top with cheese and serve.

Nutritional Value (Amount per Serving):

- Calories 568
- Fat 30.5 g
- Carbohydrates 2 g
- Sugar 0.1 g
- Protein 68.4 g
- Cholesterol 240 mg

SIMPLE DRY RUB CHICKEN WINGS

Total Time: 30 minutes

Serves: 2

Ingredients:
- 8 chicken wings
- 1/2 tsp chili powder
- 1/2 tsp garlic powder
- 1/4 tsp black pepper
- 1/4 tsp salt

Directions:
- In a bowl, mix together chili powder, garlic powder, pepper, and salt.
- Add chicken wings to the bowl and coat well with spice mixture.
- Add chicken wings into the air fryer basket and air fry at 180 C/ 356 F for 15 minutes. Shake basket halfway through.
- Cook again for 5 minutes more.
- Serve hot and enjoy.

Nutritional Value (Amount per Serving):
- Calories 84
- Fat 5.5 g
- Carbohydrates 3.7 g
- Sugar 0.2 g
- Protein 5.1 g
- Cholesterol 19 mg

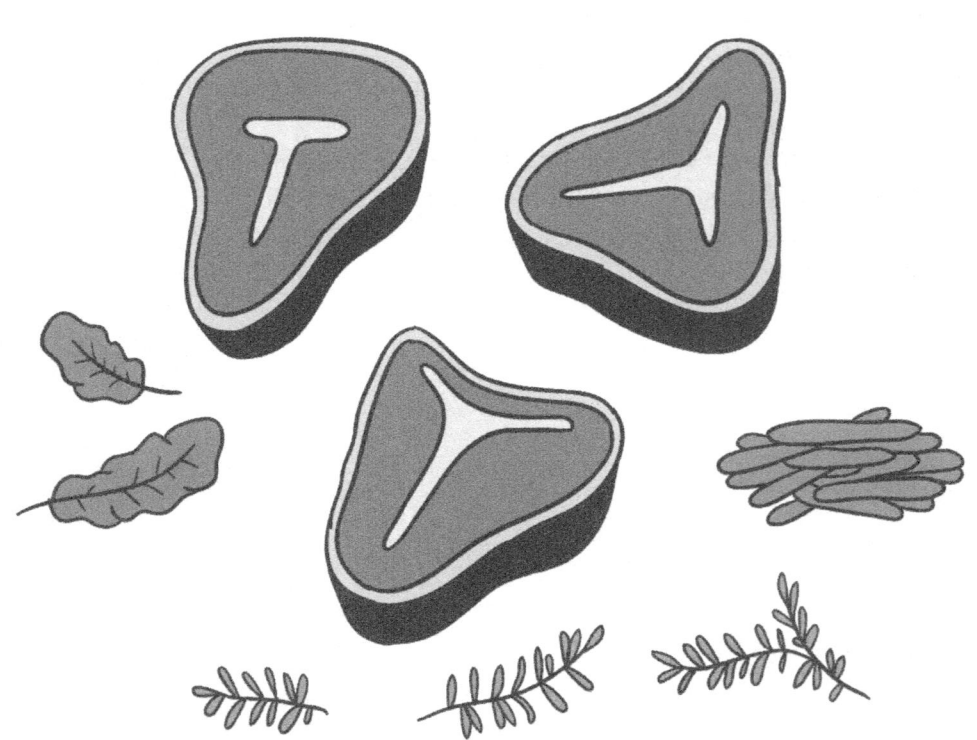

BEEF & PORK RECIPES

Contents

MONGOLIAN BEEF

Total Time: 30 minutes

Serves: 2

Ingredients:

- 1/2 lb flank steak, cut into long pieces
- 2 tbsp cornstarch
- For sauce:
- 1/4 cup brown sugar
- 1/4 cup water
- 1/4 cup soy sauce
- 1/2 tbsp garlic, minced
- 1/4 tsp ginger
- 1 tsp olive oil

Directions:

- Coat steak pieces with cornstarch and place into the air fryer basket.
- Air fry at 198 C/ 390 F for 10 minutes on each side.
- Meanwhile, for sauce add all sauce ingredients into the saucepan and heat over medium-high heat.
- Whisk sauce until starts to boil.
- Once steaks are cooked then transfer into the bowl. Pour sauce over steak and soak in about 5 minutes.
- Serve and enjoy.

Nutritional Value (Amount per Serving):

- Calories 360
- Fat 11.8 g
- Carbohydrates 28.4 g
- Sugar 18.2 g
- Protein 33.7 g
- Cholesterol 62 mg

PORK MEATBALLS

Total Time: 20 minutes

Serves: 2

Ingredients:

- 5 oz pork minced
- 1/2 tbsp fresh basil
- 1/2 onion, diced
- 1/2 tsp mustard
- 1/2 tsp honey
- 1/2 tsp garlic paste
- 1/2 tbsp cheddar cheese, grated
- Pepper
- Salt

Directions:

- Add all ingredients into the large bowl and mix well to combine.
- Make small balls from mixture and place in air fryer basket.
- Air fry pork balls at 200 C/ 392 F for 15 minutes.
- Serve and enjoy.

Nutritional Value (Amount per Serving):

- Calories 145
- Fat 7.2 g
- Carbohydrates 4.6 g
- Sugar 2.7 g
- Protein 14.5 g
- Cholesterol 2 mg

DELICIOUS MEATBALLS

Total Time: 30 minutes

Serves: 2

Ingredients:

- 1/2 lb ground lamb
- 1 egg white
- 1/2 tbsp mint, chopped
- 1 tbsp parsley, chopped
- 2 oz turkey
- 1/2 tbsp olive oil
- 1 garlic cloves, minced
- 1/2 tbsp coriander, chopped
- 1/2 tsp salt

Directions

- Preheat the air fryer to 160 C/ 320 F.
- Add all ingredients into the mixing bowl and mix well to combine.
- Make small meatballs from mixture and place in air fryer basket.
- Air fry meatballs for 15 minutes.
- Serve and enjoy.

Nutritional Value (Amount per Serving):

- Calories 301
- Fat 13.3 g
- Carbohydrates 0.9 g
- Sugar 0.2 g
- Protein 42.2 g
- Cholesterol 124 mg

BBQ PORK CHOPS

Total Time: 35 minutes

Serves: 2

Ingredients:

- 2 pork loin chops
- 1 tbsp soy sauce
- 1 garlic clove
- 1 tbsp honey
- 1/2 tsp balsamic vinegar
- 1/8 tsp ground ginger
- Pepper

Directions:

- Preheat the air fryer to 180 C/ 356 F for 5 minutes.
- Season pork chops with pepper.
- In a bowl, combine together honey, soy sauce, garlic, ground ginger, and vinegar.
- Add seasoned pork chops in a bowl and mix well and place in refrigerator for 2 hours.
- Place marinated pork chops in air fryer basket and air fry for 5 minutes on each side.
- Serve and enjoy.

Nutritional Value (Amount per Serving):

- Calories 295
- Fat 19.9 g
- Carbohydrates 9.9 g
- Sugar 8.8 g
- Protein 18.6 g
- Cholesterol 69 mg

DELICIOUS HOMEMADE BURGERS

Total Time: 20 minutes

Serves: 2

Ingredients:

- 1/2 lb ground beef
- 1/2 tsp dried parsley
- 1/4 tsp black pepper
- 1/4 tsp onion powder
- 1/4 tsp garlic powder
- 2 drops liquid smoke
- 1/2 tsp hot sauce
- 1/2 tbsp Worcestershire sauce
- 1/4 tsp salt

Directions:

- Spray air fryer basket with cooking spray.
- Add all ingredients into the large mixing bowl and mix until combined.
- Make small round patties from mixture and place into the air fryer basket.
- Cook at 180 C/ 350 F for 10 minutes.
- Serve and enjoy.

Nutritional Value (Amount per Serving):

- Calories 218
- Fat 7.1 g
- Carbohydrates 1.5 g
- Sugar 1 g
- Protein 34.5 g
- Cholesterol 101 mg

DELICIOUS STEAK

Total Time: 15 minutes

Serves: 2

Ingredients:

- 2 steaks
- 2 tsp garlic butter
- Pepper
- Salt

Directions:

- Season steaks with pepper and salt.
- Rub garlic butter over steaks.
- Place steaks into the air fryer basket and air fry at 175 C/ 350 F for 6 minutes.
- Serve and enjoy.

Nutritional Value (Amount per Serving):

- Calories 118
- Fat 8.4 g
- Carbohydrates 0 g
- Sugar 0 g
- Protein 10.4 g
- Cholesterol 7 mg

PERFECT PORK CHOPS

Total Time: 15 minutes

Serves: 2

Ingredients:

- 2 pork chops
- 1 1/2 tbsp dried parsley
- 1/4 tbsp pork seasoning
- 1 1/2 bread slices
- 1 egg
- 2 tbsp apple juice
- 1/8 tbsp olive oil
- 1.5 oz flour
- Pepper
- Salt

Directions:

- Preheat the air fryer at 175 C/ 350 F for 2 minutes.
- Blend bread slices into breadcrumbs.
- Season pork chops with pepper and salt. Rub with olive oil.
- In a large bowl, mix together flour, pork seasoning, pepper, and salt.
- In another bowl, whisk together egg and apple juice.
- In a third bowl, mix together bread crumbs, parsley, pepper, and salt.
- Coat pork chops with flour then dip into egg mixture and finally coat with breadcrumbs.
- Place pork chops into the air fryer basket and cook for 10 minutes.
- Serve and enjoy.

Nutritional Value (Amount per Serving):

- Calories 504
- Fat 23.7 g
- Carbohydrates 48 g
- Sugar 24.5 g
- Protein 23.8 g
- Cholesterol 151 mg

BUTTERY PORK CHOPS

Total Time: 20 minutes

Serves: 2

Ingredients:

- 4 pork chops
- 2 tsp parsley
- 2 tsp garlic, grated
- 1 tbsp coconut oil
- 1 tbsp coconut butter
- Pepper
- Salt

Directions:

- Preheat the air fryer to 175 C/ 347 F.
- In a large bowl, mix together garlic, butter, coconut oil, and all the seasonings.
- Rub garlic mixture into both sides of pork chops. Wrap marinated pork chops into the foil and place in the fridge for 1 hour.
- Remove pork chops from foil and place into the air fryer basket and cook for 7 minutes on one side and then turn to other side and cook for 8 minutes.
- Serve and enjoy.

Nutritional Value (Amount per Serving):

- Calories 622
- Fat 51.1 g
- Carbohydrates 2.8 g
- Sugar 0.5 g
- Protein 36.7 g
- Cholesterol 138 mg

HEALTHY BEEF BURGERS

Total Time: 25 minutes

Serves: 2

Ingredients:

- 1/2 lb ground beef
- 1 tbsp green onion, chopped
- 1/2 tbsp sesame oil
- 1 tsp sugar
- 1 tsp ginger, minced
- 1/2 tbsp soy sauce
- 1 tbsp gochujang (red chili paste)
- 1/4 tsp salt
- For mayonnaise sauce:
- 1 tbsp scallions, chopped
- 1 tsp sesame seeds
- 1/2 tbsp sesame oil
- 1/2 tbsp gochujang
- 1 tbsp mayonnaise

Directions:

- In a large bowl, mix together ground beef, onion, oil, sugar, ginger, garlic, soy sauce, gochujang, and salt. Place mixture in the fridge for 1 hour.
- Make small patties from beef mixture and place into the air fryer basket.
- Cook at 182 C/ 360 F for 10 minutes.
- In a small bowl, mix together all mayonnaise sauce ingredients.
- Serve patties with buns and mayonnaise sauce.

Nutritional Value (Amount per Serving):

- Calories 323
- Fat 17.1 g
- Carbohydrates 5.5 g
- Sugar 2.7 g
- Protein 35.2 g
- Cholesterol 103 mg

KHEEMA MEATLOAF

Total Time: 30 minutes

Serves: 2

Ingredients:

- 1 egg
- 1/2 lb ground beef
- 1/8 tsp ground cardamom
- 1/4 tsp ground cinnamon
- 1/2 tsp cayenne
- 1/2 tsp turmeric
- 1 tsp garam masala
- 1/2 tbsp garlic, minced
- 1/2 tbsp ginger, minced
- 1 tbsp cilantro, chopped
- 1/2 cup onion, chopped
- 1/2 tsp salt

Directions:

- In a large bowl, combine together all the ingredients until well mixed.
- Place meat mixture into 8 " pan and place in the air fryer basket.
- Air fry at 182 C/ 360 F for 15 minutes.
- Slice and serve.

Nutritional Value (Amount per Serving):

- Calories 266
- Fat 9.5 g
- Carbohydrates 5.5 g
- Sugar 1.5 g
- Protein 37.9 g
- Cholesterol 183 mg

AUTHENTIC BEEF SATAY

Total Time: 25 minutes

Serves: 2

Ingredients:

- 1 lb beef flank steak, sliced into long strips
- 1/4 cup peanuts, roasted and chopped
- 1/2 cup cilantro, chopped
- 1 tsp ground coriander
- 1 tsp hot sauce
- 1 tbsp sugar
- 1 tbsp garlic, minced
- 1 tbsp ginger, minced
- 1 tbsp soy sauce
- 1 tbsp fish sauce
- 2 tbsp olive oil

Directions:

- Add all ingredients except peanuts into the zip-lock bag and shake well.
- Place marinated meat into the fridge for 1 hour.
- Add marinated meat into the air fryer basket and cook at 204 C/ 400 F for 8 minutes. Turn halfway through.
- Remove meat on serving plated and garnish with roasted peanuts.
- Serve and enjoy.

Nutritional Value (Amount per Serving):

- Calories 692
- Fat 37.3 g
- Carbohydrates 13.4 g
- Sugar 7.4 g
- Protein 75.1 g
- Cholesterol 203 mg

GRILLED PORK

Total Time: 25 minutes

Serves: 2

Ingredients:

- 1/2 lb pork shoulder, cut into 1/2" slices
- 1 tbsp green onion, sliced
- 1/2 tbsp sesame seeds
- 1/4 tsp cayenne pepper
- 1/2 tsp sugar
- 1/2 tbsp sesame oil
- 1/2 tbsp rice wine
- 1/2 tbsp soy sauce
- 1/2 tbsp garlic, minced
- 1/2 tbsp ginger, minced
- 1 tbsp gochujang (red chili paste)
- 1/2 onion, sliced

Directions:

- In a large bowl, mix together all ingredients and place in the fridge for 30 minutes.
- Place pork mixture into the air fryer basket and air fry for 204 C/ 400 F for 15 minutes. Turn halfway through.
- Serve and enjoy.

Nutritional Value (Amount per Serving):

- Calories 407
- Fat 29 g
- Carbohydrates 8.2 g
- Sugar 3.4 g
- Protein 27.7 g
- Cholesterol 102 mg

JUICY KEBAB

Total Time: 20 minutes

Serves: 2

Ingredients:

- 1/2 lb ground beef
- 1 tbsp kebab spice mix
- 1/2 tbsp garlic, minced
- 1 tbsp parsley, chopped
- 1/2 tbsp olive oil
- 1/2 tsp salt

Directions:

- Add all ingredients into the stand mixer until well combined.
- Divide meat mixture into two and make two sausage shapes.
- Place kebabs into the air fryer basket and cook at 187 C/ 370 F for 10 minutes.
- Serve and enjoy.

Nutritional Value (Amount per Serving):

- Calories 244
- Fat 10.6 g
- Carbohydrates 0.8 g
- Sugar 0 g
- Protein 34.6 g
- Cholesterol 101 mg

MEATLOAF

Total Time: 35 minutes

Serves: 2

Ingredients:

- 1/2 lb ground beef
- 1 mushroom, sliced
- 1/2 tbsp fresh thyme
- 1/2 small onion, chopped
- 1 tbsp chorizo, chopped
- 1 1/2 tbsp breadcrumbs
- 1 egg, lightly beaten
- Pepper
- Salt

Directions:

- Preheat the air fryer at 204 C/ 400 F.
- In a large bowl, mix together all ingredients until well combined.
- Transfer meat mixture into the air fryer pan.
- Place pan into the air fryer basket and cook for 25 minutes.
- Slice and serve.

Nutritional Value (Amount per Serving):

- Calories 273
- Fat 9.6 g
- Carbohydrates 6.2 g
- Sugar 1.4 g
- Protein 38.4 g
- Cholesterol 183 mg

DELICIOUS BEEF MUSHROOMS MEATBALLS

Total Time: 30 minutes

Serves: 2

Ingredients:

- 1/2 lb ground beef
- 1 tbsp parsley, chopped
- 1/4 cup breadcrumbs
- 2 tbsp onion, chopped
- 1 1/2 tbsp mushrooms, diced
- 1/4 tsp pepper
- 1/2 tsp salt

Directions:

- In a mixing bowl, combine together all ingredients until well combined.
- Make small meatballs from meat mixture and place into the air fryer basket.
- Cook at 176 C/ 350 F for 20 minutes.
- Serve and enjoy.

Nutritional Value (Amount per Serving):

- Calories 270
- Fat 7.8 g
- Carbohydrates 11.1 g
- Sugar 1.3 g
- Protein 36.5 g
- Cholesterol 101 mg

BEEF FRIED RICE

Total Time: 30 minutes

Serves: 2

Ingredients:
- 1 1/2 cups rice, cooked
- 1/2 cup beef, diced
- 14 cup onion, diced
- 1/2 tbsp olive oil
- 3 tbsp soy sauce
- 1/2 cup frozen peas and carrots

Directions:
- Mix all ingredients into the air fryer pan.
- Place pan into the air fryer basket and cook at 182 C/ 360 F for 20 minutes.
- Serve warm and enjoy.

Nutritional Value (Amount per Serving):
- Calories 625
- Fat 8.2 g
- Carbohydrates 112.2 g
- Sugar 36.8 g
- Protein 31.3 g
- Cholesterol 30 mg

CHINESE PORK CHUNKS

Total Time: 30 minutes

Serves: 2

Ingredients:

- 1 egg
- 1 lb pork, cut into chunks
- 1 1/2 tbsp olive oil
- 1/8 tsp Chinese five spice
- 1/4 tsp black pepper
- 1 cup potato starch
- 1 tsp sesame oil
- 1/4 tsp salt

Directions:

- In a large bowl, combine together potato starch, Chinese five spices, pepper, and salt.
- In another bowl, whisk egg and oil.
- Dredge pork pieces into the potato starch and shake excess of if any. Now dip into the egg mixture and then return into the potato starch mixture.
- Spray air fryer basket with cooking spray.
- Place coated pork pieces into the air fryer basket.
- Cook at 171 C/ 340 F for 12 minutes.
- Serve and enjoy.

Nutritional Value (Amount per Serving):

- Calories 787
- Fat 22.9 g
- Carbohydrates 80.3 g
- Sugar 0.2 g
- Protein 62.2 g
- Cholesterol 247 mg

BBQ PORK RIBS

Total Time: 40 minutes

Serves: 2

Ingredients:

- 1 lb pork ribs
- 1 tsp soy sauce
- 1 tsp black pepper
- 1 tsp sesame oil
- 1/2 tsp five spice powder
- 1 tbsp honey
- 4 tbsp BBQ sauce
- 3 garlic cloves, chopped
- 1 tsp salt

Directions:

- Preheat the air fryer at 180 C/ 356 F for 5 minutes.
- Add all ingredients into the large bowl and m x well to coat.
- Place marinated ribs into the fridge for 1 hour.
- Add marinated ribs into the air fryer basket and air fry for 15 minutes.
- Turn ribs to other side and cook for 15 minutes more.
- Serve and enjoy.

Nutritional Value (Amount per Serving):

- Calories 729
- Fat 42.6 g
- Carbohydrates 22.4 g
- Sugar 16.9 g
- Protein 60.7 g
- Cholesterol 234 mg

STICKY PORK STRIPS

Total Time: 35 minutes

Serves: 2

Ingredients:

- 4 pork loin chops
- 1/8 tsp ground ginger
- 1 garlic clove, chopped
- 1 tbsp honey
- 1 tbsp soy sauce
- 1/2 tsp balsamic vinegar

Directions:

- Using meat tenderizers tenderize meat and season with pepper and salt.
- In a bowl, mix together honey, soy sauce, and balsamic vinegar. Add ginger and garlic and set aside.
- Add pork chops into the marinade mixture and marinate for 1 hour.
- Preheat the air fryer at 180 C/ 356 F.
- Add marinated meat into the air fryer and cook for 5-8 minutes on each side.
- Once cooked then cut into strips and serve.

Nutritional Value (Amount per Serving):

- Calories 551
- Fat 39.8 g
- Carbohydrates 9.9 g
- Sugar 8.8 g
- Protein 36.6 g
- Cholesterol 138 mg

MUSTARD HONEY PORK CHOPS

Total Time: 20 minutes

Serves: 2

Ingredients:
- 1/2 lb pork chops, boneless
- 1/2 tsp steak seasoning blend
- 1 tbsp honey
- 1/2 tbsp yellow mustard

Directions:
- In a small bowl, mix together steak seasoning, honey, and mustard.
- Brush steak seasoning mixture both side of pork chops
- Place pork chops into the air fryer basket.
- Air fry at 176 C/ 350 F for 12 minutes. Turn halfway through.
- Serve and enjoy.

Nutritional Value (Amount per Serving):
- Calories 397
- Fat 28.3 g
- Carbohydrates 8.9 g
- Sugar 8.7 g
- Protein 25.7 g
- Cholesterol 98 mg

SOUTHERN PORK CHOPS

Total Time: 25 minutes

Serves: 2

Ingredients:

- 2 pork chops, wash and pat dry
- 1/2 tsp McCormick Montreal chicken seasoning
- 2 tbsp flour
- 1 1/2 tbsp buttermilk
- Salt

Directions:

- Season pork chops with pepper and salt.
- Drizzle buttermilk over the pork chops.
- Place pork chops in a zip-lock bag with flour and shake well to coat.
- Marinate pork chops for 30 minutes.
- Place marinated pork chops into the air fryer basket and cook at 193 C/ 380 F for 15 minutes. Turn halfway through.
- Serve and enjoy.

Nutritional Value (Amount per Serving):

- Calories 289
- Fat 20.1 g
- Carbohydrates 6.5 g
- Sugar 0.6 g
- Protein 19.2 g
- Cholesterol 69 mg

BALSAMIC PORK CHOPS

Total Time: 25 minutes

Serves: 2

Ingredients:

- 1 egg
- 1/2 tbsp orange juice
- 1 tbsp raspberry jam
- 1 tbsp brown sugar
- 1/4 cup balsamic vinegar
- 2 tbsp flour
- 2 pork chops
- 1/2 cup pecans, chopped
- 1/2 cup breadcrumbs
- 2 tbsp milk
- Pepper
- Salt

Directions:

- Spray air fryer basket with cooking spray.
- Preheat the air fryer to 204 C/ 400 F.
- In a shallow bowl, whisk together milk and eggs.
- In another shallow bowl mix together pecans and breadcrumbs.
- Coat pork chops with flour then dip in egg mixture then coat with bread crumb mixture.
- Place coated pork chops into the air fryer basket and air fry for 12-15 minutes. Turn halfway through.
- For sauce: Add remaining ingredients into the small saucepan and bring to boil. Cook until thickened.
- Serve chops with sauce.

Nutritional Value (Amount per Serving):

- Calories 670
- Fat 43.9 g
- Carbohydrates 41.9 g
- Sugar 12.9 g
- Protein 28.8 g
- Cholesterol 152 mg

EASY PORK TENDERLOIN

Total Time: 25 minutes

Serves: 2

Ingredients:

- 1 pork tenderloin, cut into 4 pieces
- 1/2 tbsp mustard
- 1 tbsp oil
- 2 tsp Provencal herbs
- 1 onion, sliced
- 1 bell pepper, cut into strips
- Pepper
- Salt

Directions:

- Preheat the air fryer to 200 C/ 392 F.
- In a bowl, mix together bell pepper strips, Provencal herbs, onion, pepper, and salt. Add 1/2 tbsp oil to the mixture.
- Season pork tenderloin with mustard, pepper, and salt. Coat pork tenderloin with remaining oil.
- Place pork tenderloin pieces into the air fryer pan and top with bell pepper mixture.
- Place pan in air fryer basket and cook for 15 minutes. Turn halfway through.
- Serve and enjoy.

Nutritional Value (Amount per Serving):

- Calories 277
- Fat 11.8 g
- Carbohydrates 10.7 g
- Sugar 5.5 g
- Protein 31.6 g
- Cholesterol 83 mg

PORK LOIN WITH POTATOES

Total Time: 35 minutes

Serves: 2

Ingredients:

- 2 lb pork loin
- 1 tsp parsley, chopped
- 1/2 tsp red pepper flakes
- 1/2 tsp garlic powder
- 1 tsp pepper
- 2 potatoes, diced
- 1 tsp salt

Directions:

- Sprinkle the seasoning over the potatoes and pork loin.
- Place pork loin and potatoes into the air fryer basket and air fry at 200 C/ 392 F for 25 minutes. Turn halfway through.
- Serve and enjoy.

Nutritional Value (Amount per Serving):

- Calories 802
- Fat 16.3 g
- Carbohydrates 34.9 g
- Sugar 2.7 g
- Protein 122.6 g
- Cholesterol 331 mg

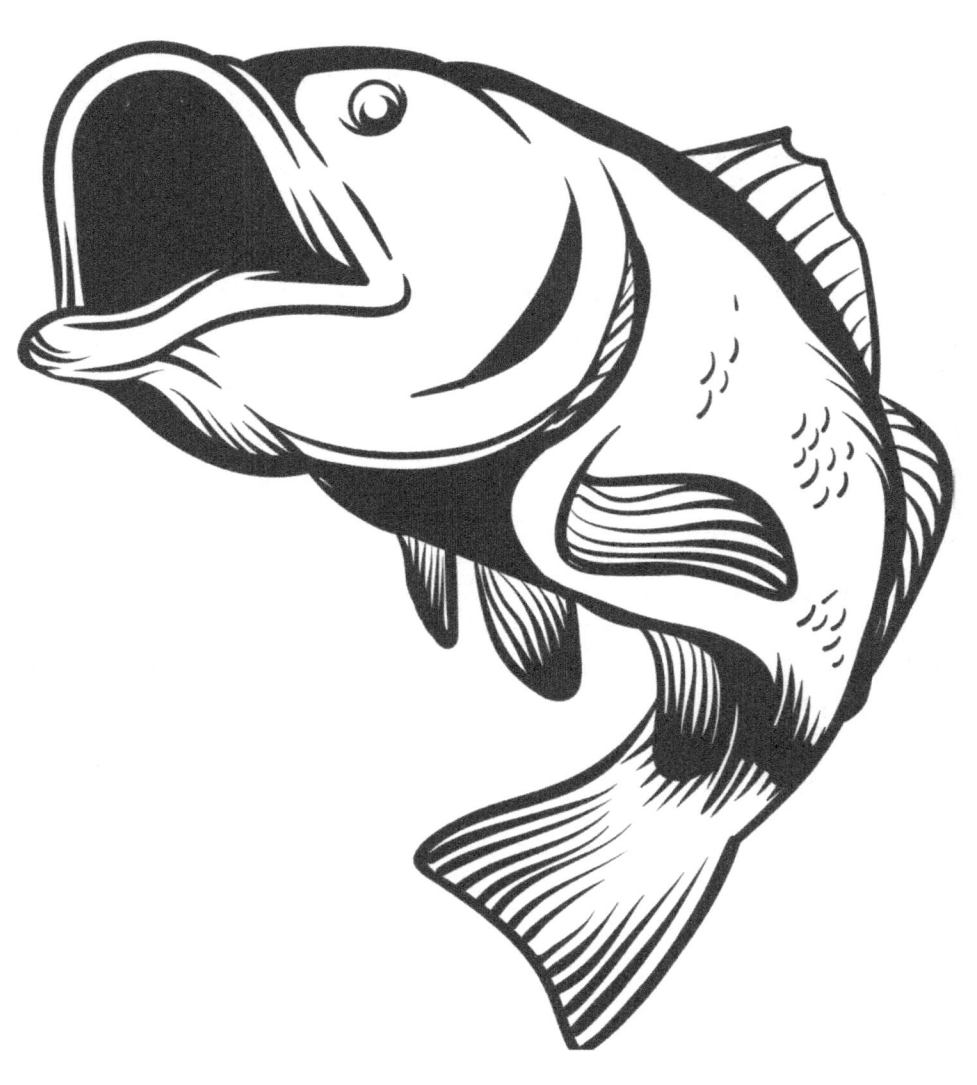

SEAFOOD RECIPES

Contents

PERFECT SALMON

Total Time: 10 minutes

Serves: 2

Ingredients:
- 2 salmon fillets, remove any bones
- 2 tsp paprika
- 2 tsp olive oil
- Pepper
- Salt

Directions:
- Rub each salmon fillet with oil, paprika, pepper, and salt.
- Place salmon fillets in the air fryer basket and air fry at 198 C/ 390 F for 7 minutes.
- Serve and enjoy.

Nutritional Value (Amount per Serving):
- Calories 282
- Fat 15.9 g
- Carbohydrates 1.2 g
- Sugar 0.2 g
- Protein 34.9 g
- Cholesterol 78 mg

RANCH FISH FILLETS

Total Time: 20 minutes

Serves: 2

Ingredients:

- 2 fish fillets
- 1 egg, lightly beaten
- 1 1/4 tbsp olive oil
- 1/2 packet ranch dressing mix
- 1/4 cup breadcrumbs

Directions:

- Preheat the air fryer to 180 C/ 356 F.
- In a shallow dish mix together ranch dressing mix and bread crumbs. Add oil and mix until mixture becomes crumbly.
- Dip fish fillet in egg then coat with bread crumb mixture and place into the air fryer basket.
- Cook for 12 minutes.
- Serve and enjoy.

Nutritional Value (Amount per Serving):

- Calories 371
- Fat 22.8 g
- Carbohydrates 25.3 g
- Sugar 1 g
- Protein 17.9 g
- Cholesterol 78 mg

CRISP FISH WITH SAUCE

Total Time: 30 minutes

Serves: 2

Ingredients:

- 2 cod fish fillets
- 1 1/4 tsp olive oil
- 1/4 cup breadcrumbs
- 1/2 tsp Dijon mustard
- 1 egg
- 2 tbsp flour
- For sauce:
- 1 tsp capers
- 1/2 tbsp tarragon, chopped
- 1/2 tbsp dill, chopped
- 1 tbsp onion, chopped
- 1 tbsp dill pickle, chopped
- 1 tbsp sour cream
- 2 tbsp mayonnaise

Directions:

- In a shallow bowl, whisk together egg and mustard.
- In another shallow dish mix together breadcrumbs and oil.
- Coat fish with flour then dip in egg mixture and finally coat with breadcrumb mixture.
- Place coated fish into the air fryer basket and cook at 180 C/ 370 F for 10 minutes.
- Meanwhile, in a small bowl, combine together all sauce ingredients.
- Serve fish with sauce and enjoy.

Nutritional Value (Amount per Serving):

- Calories 404
- Fat 13.8 g
- Carbohydrates 21 g
- Sugar 2.3 g
- Protein 47.2 g
- Cholesterol 78 mg

COCONUT SHRIMP

Total Time: 20 minutes

Serves: 2

Ingredients:

- 12 large shrimp
- 1 cup egg white
- 1 tbsp cornstarch
- 1 cup coconut, dried and unsweetened
- 1 cup flour
- 1 cup breadcrumbs

Directions

- In a shallow dish, mix together coconut and breadcrumbs and set aside.
- In another dish, mix together flour and cornstarch and set aside.
- Add egg white in a small bowl.
- Dip shrimp in egg white then coat with flour mixture and finally roll in breadcrumb mixture.
- Place coated shrimp in air fryer basket.
- Air fry shrimp at 176 C/ 350 F for 10 minutes.
- Serve and enjoy.

Nutritional Value (Amount per Serving):

- Calories 700
- Fat 17.6 g
- Carbohydrates 97.7 g
- Sugar 6.9 g
- Protein 35.8 g
- Cholesterol 69 mg

AIR FRIED TILAPIA FISH FILLET

Total Time: 20 minutes

Serves: 2

Ingredients:

- 2 tilapia fillets
- 1 tsp old bay seasoning
- 1/2 cup breadcrumbs
- 1 egg, lightly beaten
- 2 tbsp flour
- Pepper
- Salt

Directions:

- Take three small bowls. In a first bowl add flour.
- Add egg in the second's bowl and third bowl mix together bread crumbs and old bay seasoning.
- Coat fish with flour then dip in the egg and finally coat with breadcrumbs.
- Place coated fish fillets into the air fryer basket and cook for 198 C/ 390 F for 15 minutes.
- Serve and enjoy.

Nutritional Value (Amount per Serving):

- Calories 277
- Fat 6.2 g
- Carbohydrates 25.6 g
- Sugar 1.9 g
- Protein 29.2 g
- Cholesterol 132 mg

FRIED SHRIMP WITH SAUCE

Total Time: 30 minutes

Serves: 2

Ingredients:

- 1/2 lb raw shrimp, peeled and deveined
- 1/2 tsp paprika
- 1/4 cup breadcrumbs
- 1/4 cup flour
- 1 egg white
- Pepper
- Salt
- For sauce:
- 2 tbsp sweet chili sauce
- 1 tbsp sriracha
- 1/4 cup plain yogurt

Directions:

- Preheat the air fryer to 204 C/400 F.
- Season shrimp with seasoning and set aside.
- Place bread crumbs, egg whites, and flour in three separate shallow dishes.
- Now Coat shrimp with flour then dip in egg whites and finally coat with breadcrumbs.
- Spray air fryer basket with cooking spray.
- Place coated shrimp into the air fryer basket and cook for 8 minutes. Turn shrimp halfway through.
- In a small bowl, mix together all sauce ingredients.
- Serve air fried shrimp with sauce and enjoy.

Nutritional Value (Amount per Serving):

- Calories 315
- Fat 3.3 g
- Carbohydrates 33.5 g
- Sugar 9.2 g
- Protein 32.9 g
- Cholesterol 241 mg

EASY HOT PRAWNS

Total Time: 25 minutes

Serves: 2

Ingredients:

- 6 prawns
- 1/2 tsp chili powder
- 1 tsp chili flakes
- 1/4 tsp black pepper
- 1/4 tsp salt

Directions:

- Preheat the air fryer to 180 C/356 F.
- In a bowl, mix together spices add prawns to the bowl and toss well with spices.
- Spray air fryer basket with cooking spray.
- Transfer prawns to the air fryer basket and cook for 6-8 minutes.
- Serve and enjoy.

Nutritional Value (Amount per Serving):

- Calories 81
- Fat 1.2 g
- Carbohydrates 1.6 g
- Sugar 0.1 g
- Protein 15.2 g
- Cholesterol 139 mg

DELICIOUS SCALLOPS

Total Time: 30 minutes

Serves: 2

Ingredients:

- 8 sea scallops
- 12 oz frozen spinach, thawed and drained
- 1 tsp garlic, minced
- 1 tbsp fresh basil, chopped
- 1 tbsp tomato paste
- 3/4 cup heavy whipping cream
- 1/2 tsp pepper
- 1/2 tsp salt

Directions:

- Spray 7" pan with cooking spray. Layer spinach in the pan.
- Spray scallops with cooking spray and season with pepper and salt.
- Place scallops into the pan on top of spinach.
- In a small bowl, mix together garlic, basil, tomato paste, whipping cream, pepper, and salt and pour over scallops and spinach.
- Place pan into the air fryer and cook at 176 C/350 F for 10 minutes.
- Serve hot and enjoy.

Nutritional Value (Amount per Serving):

- Calories 310
- Fat 18.3 g
- Carbohydrates 12.6 g
- Sugar 1.7 g
- Protein 26.5 g
- Cholesterol 101 mg

FLAVORFUL FISH PACKETS

Total Time: 25 minutes

Serves: 2

Ingredients:

- 2 cod fish fillets
- 1 tbsp olive oil
- 1 tbsp lemon juice
- 2 pats butter, melted
- 1/2 tsp dried tarragon
- 1/2 cup red peppers, sliced
- 1/4 cup celery, cut into julienne
- 1/2 cup carrots, cut into julienne
- Pepper
- Salt

Directions:

- In a bowl, combine together butter, lemon juice, tarragon, and salt. Add vegetables and mix well. Set aside.
- Take two parchments paper pieces to hold fish and vegetables.
- Spray fish with cooking spray and season with pepper and salt.
- Place a fish fillet on each parchment paper piece and top each fillet with vegetables.
- Fold parchment paper and crimp all the sides to hold the vegetables and fish.
- Place fish vegetable packets into the air fryer basket and cook at 176 C/350 F for 15 minutes.
- Serve and enjoy.

Nutritional Value (Amount per Serving):

- Calories 280
- Fat 8.8 g
- Carbohydrates 6.7 g
- Sugar 3.7 g
- Protein 42.2 g
- Cholesterol 99 mg

CREAMY SPICY CRAB DIP

Total Time: 15 minutes

Serves: 2

Ingredients:

- 1/2 cup crab, cooked
- 1 tbsp parsley, chopped
- 1 tbsp lemon juice
- 1/2 tsp pepper
- 1 tbsp hot sauce
- 1/4 cup scallions
- 1 cup cheese, grated
- 1 tbsp mayonnaise
- 1/4 tsp salt

Directions:

- In a 6" dish, mix together cooked crab, hot sauce, scallions, cheese, mayonnaise, pepper, and salt.
- Place dish into the air fryer basket.
- Cook at 204 C/400 F for 7 minutes.
- Remove pan from air fryer. Add parsley and lemon juice. Mix well.
- Serve hot and enjoy.

Nutritional Value (Amount per Serving):

- Calories 295
- Fat 21.8 g
- Carbohydrates 4.2 g
- Sugar 1.3 g
- Protein 20.6 g
- Cholesterol 91 mg

SALMON WITH VEGGIES

Total Time: 30 minutes

Serves: 2

Ingredients:

- 2 salmon fillets
- 1 tbsp olive oil
- 3 tbsp rice wine vinegar
- 1/4 cup soy sauce
- 1/2 cup orange juice
- 2 tsp orange zest
- 1 tbsp ginger, minced
- 2 garlic cloves, minced
- 1/2 tsp salt
- For veggies:
- 2 heads baby Bok Choy
- 1 tbsp sesame oil
- 2 oz mushrooms, remove stems
- Salt

Directions:

- In a small bowl, mix together garlic, olive oil, vinegar, soy sauce, orange juice, orange zest, ginger, and salt.
- Place salmon in zip-lock bag and pour half garlic mixture over the salmon. Seal bag and massage to coat well.
- Allow to marinate for 40 minutes.
- Place marinated salmon in air fryer basket and cook at 204 C/400 F for 6 minutes.
- Meanwhile, brush mushroom and Bok Choy with sesame oil and season with salt.
- Once 6 minutes over then add vegetables around the salmon and cook continue for 6 minutes,
- Drizzle salmon with remaining garlic mixture and serve.

Nutritional Value (Amount per Serving):

- Calories 547
- Fat 26.9 g
- Carbohydrates 31.5 g
- Sugar 16.3 g
- Protein 50.9 g
- Cholesterol 78 mg

TASTY MAYO SHRIMP

Total Time: 15 minutes

Serves: 2

Ingredients:
- 1/2 lb shrimp, peeled
- 1/4 tsp paprika
- 1/2 tsp sriracha
- 1/2 tbsp garlic, minced
- 1/2 tbsp ketchup
- 1 1/2 tbsp mayonnaise
- 1/4 tsp salt

Directions:
- In a bowl, mix together mayonnaise, paprika, sriracha, garlic, ketchup, and salt.
- Add shrimp into the bowl and coat well with sauce.
- Spray air fryer basket with cooking spray and place shrimp into the basket.
- Cook at 162 C/ 325 F for 8 minutes. Shake halfway through.
- Serve and enjoy.

Nutritional Value (Amount per Serving):
- Calories 187
- Fat 5.7 g
- Carbohydrates 6.4 g
- Sugar 1.6 g
- Protein 26.2 g
- Cholesterol 242 mg

DELICIOUS CRAB CAKES

Total Time: 25 minutes

Serves: 2

Ingredients:

- 3/4 cup crabmeat, drained
- 1/4 cup breadcrumbs
- 18 tsp wasabi
- 1 1/2 tbsp mayonnaise
- 1 large egg whites
- 2 green onions, chopped
- 1/2 celery rib, chopped
- 1/2 medium sweet red pepper, chopped
- 1/8 tsp salt

Directions:

- Preheat the air fryer 190 C/ 375 F.
- Spray air fryer basket with cooking spray.
- Place bread crumbs in a shallow bowl.
- In a bowl, add remaining ingredients except for crab and mix well. Gently fold in crabmeat.
- Drop a tablespoon of crabmeat mixture to the breadcrumbs and slowly coat and shape into patties.
- Place crab cakes into the air fryer basket and cook for 10-12 minutes. Turn halfway through.
- Serve and enjoy.

Nutritional Value (Amount per Serving):

- Calories 146
- Fat 4.7 g
- Carbohydrates 21.6 g
- Sugar 3.5 g
- Protein 5.4 g
- Cholesterol 3 mg

BROILED FISH FILLETS

Total Time: 15 minutes

Serves: 2

Ingredients:

- 2 tilapia fillets
- 1/2 tsp butter
- 1/4 tsp lemon pepper
- 1/2 tsp old bay seasoning
- Pepper
- Salt

Directions:

- Spray air fryer basket with cooking spray.
- Place fish fillets in the air fryer basket and season with spices and salt.
- Spray fish fillets with cooking spray.
- Cook at 204 C/400 F for 7 minutes.
- Serve and enjoy.

Nutritional Value (Amount per Serving):

- Calories 79
- Fat 2 g
- Carbohydrates 0.2 g
- Sugar 0 g
- Protein 16.1 g
- Cholesterol 45 mg

MISO FISH

Total Time: 20 minutes

Serves: 2

Ingredients:
- 2 cod fish fillets
- 1 tbsp garlic, chopped
- 2 tbsp brown sugar
- 2 tbsp miso

Directions:
- Add all ingredients to the zip-lock bag and marinate fish in the refrigerator for overnight.
- Preheat the air fryer at 200 C/ 392 F for 2 minutes.
- Set air fryer to 180 C/ 356 F and place marinated fish fillets into the air fryer basket and air fry for 10 minutes.
- Serve and enjoy.

Nutritional Value (Amount per Serving):
- Calories 264
- Fat 2.6 g
- Carbohydrates 14.8 g
- Sugar 9.8 g
- Protein 43.4 g
- Cholesterol 99 mg

HEALTHY SHRIMP VEGETABLES

Total Time: 25 minutes

Serves: 2

Ingredients:

- 25 small shrimp, peeled and deveined
- 1/2 tbsp Cajun seasoning
- 1/2 bag frozen mix vegetables

Directions:

- Add vegetables and shrimp into the air fryer basket and sprinkle with seasoning.
- Spray shrimp and vegetables with cooking spray.
- Cook at 179 C/ 355 F for 10 minutes.
- Open air fryer basket and mix well and continue cooking for 10 minutes more.
- Serve and enjoy.

Nutritional Value (Amount per Serving):

- Calories 48
- Fat 0.2 g
- Carbohydrates 9 g
- Sugar 2.2 g
- Protein 2.6 g
- Cholesterol 4 mg

VEGETARIAN RECIPES

Contents

DELICIOUS CHILI HONEY POTATOES

Total Time: 30 minutes

Serves: 2

Ingredients:

- 1 large potato, peeled and cut in fries shape
- 1 tbsp fresh parsley, chopped
- 1 tbsp olive oil
- 1 1/2 tbsp corn flour
- Pepper
- Salt
- For sauce:

- 1/2 tbsp red chili flakes
- 1/2 tsp soy sauce
- 1 1/2 tbsp honey
- 2 tbsp tomato ketchup
- 1 tbsp garlic, chopped
- 1 tbsp butter
- Pepper
- Salt

Directions:

- Preheat the air fryer to 356 F/ 180 C for 10 minutes.
- In a bowl, mix together potatoes, corn flour, olive oil, pepper, and salt.
- Add potato fries in the preheated air fryer basket and cook for 15 minutes or until lightly golden.
- Meanwhile, add all sauce ingredients in a pan and boil over medium-high heat for 2 minutes.
- Transfer potato fries in a mixing bowl. Pour sauce over potato fries and mix well.
- Garnish with chopped parsley and serve.

Nutritional Value (Amount per Serving):

- Calories 343
- Fat 13.2 g
- Carbohydrates 54.9 g
- Sugar 17.9 g
- Protein 4.9 g
- Cholesterol 15 mg

ROASTED CORN

Total Time: 15 minutes

Serves: 2

Ingredients:

- 2 fresh ears of corn, remove husks, wash, and pat dry
- 2 tsp oil
- 1 tbsp fresh lemon juice
- Pepper
- Salt

Directions:

- Cut the corn to fit in air fryer basket.
- Drizzle oil over the corn. Season with pepper and salt.
- Cook at 204 C/ 400 F for 10 minutes.
- Sprinkle fresh lemon juice over corn and serve.

Nutritional Value (Amount per Serving):

- Calories 174
- Fat 6.4 g
- Carbohydrates 29.2 g
- Sugar 5.2 g
- Protein 5.1 g
- Cholesterol 0 mg

POTATO KALE NUGGETS

Total Time: 25 minutes

Serves: 2

Ingredients:

- 1 cup potatoes, boiled, peeled and chopped
- 1 tbsp almond milk
- 2 cups kale, chopped
- 1 garlic clove, minced
- 1 tsp olive oil
- Pepper
- Salt

Directions:

- Heat oil in a pan over medium-high heat.
- Add garlic and sauté until lightly brown. Add kale and sauté for 2-3 minutes. Transfer to the mixing bowl.
- In another bowl, add boiled potatoes, almond milk, pepper, and salt and mash with potato masher.
- Transfer potato mixture to the mixing bowl and mix well with kale.
- Preheat the air fryer 198 C/ 390 F for 5 minutes.
- Roll the kale and potato mixture into the small nuggets.
- Spray air fryer basket with cooking spray and place prepared nuggets in the basket.
- Cook nuggets in preheated air fryer for 10-12 minutes or until lightly golden brown. Shake basket halfway through.
- Serve and enjoy.

Nutritional Value (Amount per Serving):

- Calories 124
- Fat 4.2 g
- Carbohydrates 19.7 g
- Sugar 1.1 g
- Protein 3.5 g
- Cholesterol 0 mg

VEGAN TOFU

Total Time: 35 minutes

Serves: 2

Ingredients:

- 1/2 lb tofu, drained, pressed and cut into cubes
- 1/2 tbsp cornstarch
- 1/2 tbsp tamari
- For sauce:
- 1/2 tbsp maple syrup
- 1/2 tsp garlic, minced
- 1/2 tsp ginger, minced
- 1/8 tsp red pepper flakes
- 1 tsp cornstarch
- 1/4 cup water
- 1/4 cup orange juice
- 1/2 tsp orange zest

Directions:

- Add tofu and tamari into the zip-lock bag. Seal bag and shake well to coat tofu with tamari.
- Add 1/2 tablespoon of cornstarch to the zip-lock bag and shake again. Set aside for 15 minutes.
- Meanwhile, In a small bowl, mix together all sauce ingredients and set aside.
- Place marinated tofu cube in air fryer basket and cook for 198 C/ 390 F for 10 minutes. Shake halfway through.
- Add air fried tofu to a pan over medium-high heat. Pour sauce over tofu and stir well and cook until sauce thickened.
- Serve hot and enjoy.

Nutritional Value (Amount per Serving):

- Calories 125
- Fat 4.9 g
- Carbohydrates 12.5 g
- Sugar 6.4 g
- Protein 10.1 g
- Cholesterol 0 mg

VEGETABLE FRITTERS

Total Time: 25 minutes

Serves: 2

Ingredients:

- 1 1/2 cups frozen vegetable
- 1/4 tsp olive oil
- 1/4 tsp garlic powder
- 1/4 cup parmesan cheese, shredded
- 1/2 tbsp coconut flour
- 1 egg, lightly beaten
- Pepper
- Salt

Directions:

- Steam frozen vegetables and mash vegetables in a bowl. Allow to cool.
- Add egg in mash vegetables and stir well.
- Add parmesan cheese, coconut flour, garlic powder, pepper, and salt and stir well.
- Coat air fryer basket with olive oil.
- Make small patties from the mixture and arrange in the air fryer basket.
- Cook at 198 C/ 390 F for 15 minutes. Turn halfway through.
- Serve and enjoy.

Nutritional Value (Amount per Serving):

- Calories 183
- Fat 6.2 g
- Carbohydrates 20.7 g
- Sugar 4.8 g
- Protein 11 g
- Cholesterol 89 mg

DELICIOUS POTATO WEDGES

Total Time: 30 minutes

Serves: 2

Ingredients:

- 1/2 lb potatoes, cut into wedges
- 1/4 tsp garlic powder
- 1/2 tsp olive oil
- 1/2 tsp pepper
- 1/2 tsp salt
- For sauce:
- 1/4 cup water
- 1/2 tsp lemon juice
- 1 tbsp nutritional yeast
- 1/4 tsp paprika
- 1/4 tsp turmeric
- 1/4 cup raw cashews

Directions:

- Preheat the air fryer to 204 C/ 400 F for 3 minutes.
- Add potato wedges into the large bowl. Add garlic powder, pepper, salt, and oil and toss well to coat.
- Transfer potato wedges to the air fryer basket and air fry for 15 minutes. Shake halfway through.
- Add all sauce ingredients to the blender and blend until you get a thick consistency.
- Transfer air fried potato wedges to the air fryer safe pan and drizzle with prepared sauce over the potato wedges.
- Place pan in the air fryer and cook for 2 minutes more.
- Serve and enjoy.

Nutritional Value (Amount per Serving):

- Calories 209
- Fat 9.6 g
- Carbohydrates 26.7 g
- Sugar 2.3 g
- Protein 7 g
- Cholesterol 0 mg

PERFECT BRUSSELS SPROUTS

Total Time: 20 minutes

Serves: 2

Ingredients:
- 1/2 lb Brussels sprouts, rinse and pat dry with a paper towel
- 1/2 tsp garlic powder
- 1 tbsp lemon juice
- 1/4 tsp black pepper
- 1 tbsp olive oil
- 1/2 tsp salt

Directions:
- Cut the stem of Brussels sprouts and cut each Brussels sprouts in half.
- Transfer Brussels sprouts in a bowl and toss with garlic powder, olive oil, pepper, and salt.
- Transfer Brussels sprouts to the air fryer basket and cook at 182 C/ 360 F for 12 minutes. Shake basket halfway through.
- Transfer to the serving plate and drizzle with lemon juice.
- Serve and enjoy.

Nutritional Value (Amount per Serving):
- Calories 114
- Fat 7.5 g
- Carbohydrates 11.2 g
- Sugar 2.8 g
- Protein 4.1 g
- Cholesterol 0 mg

TARO FRIES

Total Time: 25 minutes

Serves: 2

Ingredients:

- 8 small taro, peel and slice like French fries
- 1/2 tsp salt
- 1 tbsp olive oil

Directions:

- Add taro slice in a bowl and toss well with olive oil and salt.
- Transfer taro slices to the air fryer basket and cook at 180 C/ 360 F for 20 minutes. Toss halfway through.
- Serve and enjoy.

Nutritional Value (Amount per Serving):

- Calories 118
- Fat 7.1 g
- Carbohydrates 13.8 g
- Sugar 0.2 g
- Protein 0.8 g
- Cholesterol 0 mg

STIR FRIED CAULIFLOWER

Total Time: 30 minutes

Serves: 2

Ingredients:

- 1/2 cauliflower head, cut into florets
- 1 scallion, chopped
- 1/2 tbsp hot sauce
- 1/4 tsp coconut sugar
- 1/2 tbsp rice vinegar
- 3/4 tbsp tamari
- 2 garlic cloves, sliced
- 1/4 cup onion, sliced

Directions:

- Place cauliflower florets into the air fryer basket.
- Cook at 176 C/ 350 F for 10 minutes.
- Remove air fryer basket and shake well. Add onion and cook for 10 minutes more.
- Add garlic and stir well and cook for 5 minutes.
- In a small bowl, mix together soy sauce, hot sauce, coconut sugar, vinegar, pepper, and salt.
- Pour soy sauce mixture over cauliflower and stir well and cook for 5 minutes more.
- Garnish with scallions and serve.

Nutritional Value (Amount per Serving):

- Calories 38
- Fat 0.1 g
- Carbohydrates 7.3 g
- Sugar 3.1 g
- Protein 2.5 g
- Cholesterol 0 mg

MUSHROOM RICE

Total Time: 25 minutes

Serves: 2

Ingredients:

- 5.3 oz jasmine rice, rinsed and drained
- 3 tbsp frozen peas
- 5.3 oz cremini mushrooms, clean and cut
- 1 1/4 tbsp white wine
- 1/4 tsp ginger powder
- 3/4 tsp 5 spice powder
- 2 garlic cloves, chopped
- 1 1/4 tbsp maple syrup
- 1 tbsp soy sauce

Directions:

- Cook rice according to the packet directions.
- In a small bowl, mix together soy sauce, maple syrup, garlic, spice powder, and ground ginger. Set aside.
- Place mushroom in air fryer and cook at 176 C/ 350 F for 10 minutes. Shake halfway through.
- Open air fryer basket and pour soy sauce mixture and peas over the mushroom. Stir well and cook for 5 minutes more.
- Pour mushroom mixture over cooked rice.
- Stir well and serve.

Nutritional Value (Amount per Serving):

- Calories 82
- Fat 0.2 g
- Carbohydrates 15.6 g
- Sugar 9.7 g
- Protein 3.4 g
- Cholesterol 0 mg

CRISP AVOCADO FRIES

Total Time: 20 minutes

Serves: 2

Ingredients:

- 1 large avocado, peeled, pitted and sliced
- 1/2 cup breadcrumbs
- 1 egg, lightly beaten
- 1/2 tsp sea salt

Directions

- Take two shallow dishes.
- Mix together breadcrumbs and salt in one dish.
- Add beaten egg in the second dish.
- Dip avocado slice into the beaten egg then coats with breadcrumbs.
- Place coated avocado slices in air fryer basket.
- Air fry at 198C/390 F for 10 minutes. Turn halfway through.
- Serve and enjoy.

Nutritional Value (Amount per Serving):

- Calories 168
- Fat 6.1 g
- Carbohydrates 21.1 g
- Sugar 1.8 g
- Protein 6.9 g
- Cholesterol 82 mg

DELICIOUS CRISP OKRA

Total Time: 30 minutes

Serves: 2

Ingredients:

- 3 cups okra, wash and dry
- 1 tsp red chili powder
- 3 tbsp gram flour
- 1/2 tsp coriander powder
- 1 tsp cumin powder
- 1 tsp dry mango powder
- 1 tsp fresh lemon juice
- Salt

Directions

- Preheat the air fryer to 200 C/392 F for 5 minutes.
- Cut top of okra then makes a deep horizontal cut in each okra and set aside.
- In a bowl, combine together gram flour, lemon juice, chili powder, coriander powder, cumin powder, mango powder, and salt.
- Add little water in gram flour mixture and make a thick batter.
- Fill batter in each okra and place in air fryer basket.
- Spray okra with cooking spray.
- Air fry stuffed okra for 10 minutes.
- Serve and enjoy.

Nutritional Value (Amount per Serving):

- Calories 102
- Fat 1.3 g
- Carbohydrates 17.4 g
- Sugar 3.3 g
- Protein 5.2 g
- Cholesterol 0 mg

AIR-FRIED MUSHROOMS

Total Time: 40 minutes

Serves: 2

Ingredients:

- 1 lbs mushrooms, wash, dry and cut into quarter
- 1/4 tsp garlic powder
- 1/2 tbsp olive oil
- 1 tbsp white vermouth
- 1 tsp herb de Provence

Directions

- Add all ingredients to the bowl and toss well.
- Transfer mushrooms into the air fryer basket.
- Air fry mushrooms at 180 C/ 356 F for 25 minutes. Shake basket twice.
- Serve and enjoy.

Nutritional Value (Amount per Serving):

- Calories 80
- Fat 4.2 g
- Carbohydrates 7.7 g
- Sugar 4 g
- Protein 7.2 g
- Cholesterol 0 mg

CRISP BROCCOLI FLORETS

Total Time: 30 minutes

Serves: 2

Ingredients:

- 1 lb broccoli florets
- 2 tbsp plain yogurt
- 1 tbsp chickpea flour
- 1/2 tsp chili powder
- 1/4 tsp turmeric powder
- 1/2 tsp salt

Directions

- Add all ingredients to the bowl and toss well.
- Place marinated broccoli in a refrigerator for 15 minutes.
- Preheat the air fryer to 200 C/ 392 F.
- Place marinated broccoli into the air fryer basket and air fry for 10 minutes. Shake basket halfway through.
- Serve and enjoy.

Nutritional Value (Amount per Serving):

- Calories 114
- Fat 1.5 g
- Carbohydrates 20.5 g
- Sugar 5.7 g
- Protein 8.5 g
- Cholesterol 1 mg

EASY ZUCCHINI FRIES

Total Time: 20 minutes

Serves: 2

Ingredients:

- 2 medium zucchini, cut into French fries shape
- 2 tbsp cornstarch
- 1 tbsp water
- 1/2 tbsp olive oil
- Salt

Directions

- Preheat the air fryer at 198 C/390 F.
- Add all ingredients into the bowl and mix well.
- Place coated zucchini fries in air fryer basket and air fry for 15 minutes.
- Serve and enjoy.

Nutritional Value (Amount per Serving):

- Calories 92
- Fat 3.9 g
- Carbohydrates 13.9 g
- Sugar 3.4 g
- Protein 2.4 g
- Cholesterol 0 mg

CASHEW ROAST

Total Time: 15 minutes

Serves: 2

Ingredients:

- 3/4 cups cashews
- 1/2 tsp olive oil
- 1/4 tsp black pepper
- 1/2 tsp chili powder
- 1/2 tsp coriander powder
- 1/4 tsp salt

Directions

- Add all ingredients into the bowl and toss we l.
- Add cashews in air fryer basket and air fry at 120 C/248 F for 10 minutes.
- Allow to cool completely then serve.

Nutritional Value (Amount per Serving):

- Calories 308
- Fat 25.1 g
- Carbohydrates 17.3 g
- Sugar 2.6 g
- Protein 8 g
- Cholesterol 0 mg

DESSERTS RECIPES

Contents

CINNAMON PINEAPPLE SLICES

Total Time: 45 minutes

Serves: 2

Ingredients:

- 4 pineapple slices
- 1 tsp cinnamon
- 1/2 cup brown sugar

Directions:

- Add cinnamon and brown sugar in a zip-lock bag and mix well.
- Add pineapple slices in the zip-lock bag and shake well to coat with cinnamon and brown sugar.
- Seal bag and place in refrigerator for 20 minutes.
- Preheat the air fryer to 180 C/ 356 F.
- Place pineapple slices on air fryer wire rack.
- Grill pineapple slices for 10 minutes then turn to another side and grill for 10 minutes more.
- Serve and enjoy.

Nutritional Value (Amount per Serving):

- Calories 156
- Fat 0 g
- Carbohydrates 40.5 g
- Sugar 38.7 g
- Protein 0.1 g
- Cholesterol 0 mg

CHOCOLATE SOUFFLÉ

Total Time: 30 minutes

Serves: 2

Ingredients:

- 2 eggs, separated
- 2 tbsp all purpose flour
- 1/2 tsp vanilla extract
- 3 tbsp sugar
- 1/4 cup butter
- 3 oz chocolate, chopped

Directions:

- Spray two ramekins with cooking spray and set aside.
- Melt butter and chocolate in a double boiler and set aside.
- In a bowl, beat together sugar, egg yolks, and vanilla. Drizzle in butter and chocolate. Mix well.
- Add flour and mix until no lumps.
- Preheat the air fryer at 165 C/ 330 F.
- In a separate bowl, beat egg whites until soft peaks form.
- Add 1/3 of egg whites to the chocolate mixture and mix slowly, until all the egg whites combine with chocolate mixture.
- Pour batter into the prepared ramekins. Place ramekins into the air fryer basket and cook for 14 minutes.
- Serve and enjoy.

Nutritional Value (Amount per Serving):

- Calories 593
- Fat 40.1 g
- Carbohydrates 49.7 g
- Sugar 40.4 g
- Protein 9.8 g
- Cholesterol 234 mg

CHOCOLATE MUG CAKE

Total Time: 15 minutes

Serves: 2

Ingredients:

- 6 tsp coconut oil
- 6 tbsp milk
- 2 tbsp cocoa powder
- 10 tbsp caster sugar
- 1/2 cup self-raising flour

Directions:

- Add all ingredients to the mixing bowl and mix until well combined.
- Divide mixture into the two cups.
- Place cups in air fryer and cook at 392 F/ 200 C for 10 minutes.
- Serve and enjoy.

Nutritional Value (Amount per Serving):

- Calories 491
- Fat 15.6 g
- Carbohydrates 89.1 g
- Sugar 62.2 g
- Protein 5.7 g
- Cholesterol 4 mg

LAVA CAKES

Total Time: 25 minutes

Serves: 2

Ingredients:

- 1 egg
- 1.75 oz dark chocolate, chopped
- 1.75 oz butter
- 1.75 tbsp sugar
- 3/4 tbsp self-rising flour

Directions:

- Preheat the air fryer at 190 C/ 375 F.
- Spray 2 ramekins with cooking spray and set aside.
- Melt butter and dark chocolate in microwave safe bowl for 2-3 minutes. Remove from microwave and stir well.
- In a separate bowl, beat sugar and egg until frothy.
- Pour chocolate mixture into the egg mixture. Add flour and stir everything well.
- Pour batter into the prepared ramekins and bake in preheated air fryer for 10 minutes.
- Remove ramekins from air fryer and allow to cool for 2 minutes. Turn ramekins upside down onto the plate.
- Serve immediately and enjoy.

Nutritional Value (Amount per Serving):

- Calories 392
- Fat 29.7 g
- Carbohydrates 27.7 g
- Sugar 23.5 g
- Protein 5.2 g
- Cholesterol 141 mg

BRAZILIAN GRILLED PINEAPPLE WEDGES

Total Time: 20 minutes

Serves: 2

Ingredients:

- 1/2 small pineapple, peeled, cored and cut into wedges
- 1 1/2 tbsp butter, melted
- 1 tsp cinnamon
- 1/4 cup brown sugar

Directions:

- In a small bowl, mix together cinnamon and sugar.
- Brush pineapple wedges with butter and sprinkle with brown sugar mixture.
- Place pineapple wedges into the air fryer basket and air fry at 204 C/ 400 F for 10 minutes.
- Serve and enjoy.

Nutritional Value (Amount per Serving):

- Calories 271
- Fat 9 g
- Carbohydrates 51.2 g
- Sugar 42 g
- Protein 1.5 g
- Cholesterol 23 mg

BLUEBERRY MUFFINS

Total Time: 25 minutes

Serves: 2

Ingredients:

- 1 egg
- 3/4 cup blueberries
- 3 tbsp butter, melted
- 1/3 cup milk
- 2 tbsp sugar
- 1 tsp baking powder
- 2/3 cup flour

Directions:

- Spray four silicone muffins cups with cooking spray and set aside.
- In a bowl, mix together all ingredients until well combined.
- Pour batter into the prepared muffins cups.
- Place muffin cups in air fryer basket and cook at 160 C/ 320 F for 14 minutes.
- Serve and enjoy.

Nutritional Value (Amount per Serving):

- Calories 435
- Fat 20.9 g
- Carbohydrates 55 g
- Sugar 19.5 g
- Protein 9 g
- Cholesterol 131 mg

SWEET NUTELLA SANDWICH

Total Time: 15 minutes

Serves: 2

Ingredients:

- 4 bread slices
- 1 banana, cut in half and slice each half in 3 slices
- 1/4 cup Nutella
- 1 tbsp butter, softened

Directions:

- Preheat the air fryer to 187 C/ 370 F.
- Spread butter on one side of each bread slices and place butter side down.
- Spread Nutella on another side of each bread slices.
- Place banana slices on 2 bread slices and top with remaining bread slices.
- Cut the sandwiches in half and place in an air fryer basket.
- Cook in preheated air fryer for 5 minutes. Turn sandwiches after 2 minutes.
- Serve and enjoy.

Nutritional Value (Amount per Serving):

- Calories 341
- Fat 18.5 g
- Carbohydrates 42.6 g
- Sugar 27 g
- Protein 4.3 g
- Cholesterol 15 mg

VEGAN BROWNIES

Total Time: 30 minutes

Serves: 2

Ingredients:

- 1/4 cup whole wheat pastry flour
- 1/2 tbsp ground flax seeds
- 2 tbsp cocoa powder
- 1/4 cup vegan sugar
- 1/8 tsp salt
- Wet ingredients:
- 1/4 tsp vanilla
- 2 tbsp aquafaba
- 2 tbsp almond milk

Directions:

- Preheat the air fryer at 176 C/ 350 F.
- Spray pie round pan with cooking spray and set aside.
- In a bowl, mix together all dry ingredients.
- Add wet ingredients to dry ingredients and mix well to combine.
- Pour batter to the prepared pan and place in air fryer basket.
- Cook in preheated air fryer for 20 minutes.
- Cut into pieces and serve.

Nutritional Value (Amount per Serving):

- Calories 202
- Fat 5.1 g
- Carbohydrates 39.4 g
- Sugar 24.7 g
- Protein 3.1 g
- Cholesterol 0 mg

GLUTEN FREE CHOCÓ LAVA CAKE

Total Time: 15 minutes

Serves: 2

Ingredients:

- 1 egg
- 1/2 tsp baking powder
- 1 tbsp coconut oil, melted
- 1 tbsp flax meal
- 1/8 tsp stevia
- 2 tbsp erythritol
- 2 tbsp water
- 2 tbsp cocoa powder
- 1/8 tsp vanilla
- Pinch of salt

Directions:

- Spray two ramekins with cooking spray and set aside.
- Add all ingredients to the bowl and whisk well.
- Preheat the air fryer to 176 C/ 350 F for a minute.
- Pour batter into the prepared ramekins. Place ramekins into the air fryer basket and cook for 8-9 minutes.
- Serve warm and enjoy.

Nutritional Value (Amount per Serving):

- Calories 122
- Fat 11 g
- Carbohydrates 17 g
- Sugar 0.3 g
- Protein 4.5 g
- Cholesterol 82 mg

WALNUT BANANA MUFFINS

Total Time: 20 minutes

Serves: 2

Ingredients:

- 4 tbsp flour
- 1/2 tsp baking powder
- 1/4 cup powdered sugar
- 1/4 cup butter
- 1/4 cup banana, mashed
- 1/4 cup oats
- 1 tbsp walnuts, chopped

Directions:

- Spray four muffin molds with cooking spray and set aside.
- In a bowl, mix together mashed banana, walnuts, sugar, and butter.
- In another bowl, mix together flour, baking powder, and oats.
- Add flour mixture to the banana mixture and mix well.
- Pour batter into the prepared muffin mold. Place air fryer basket and cook at 160 C/ 320 F for 10 minutes.
- Remove muffins from air fryer and allow to cool completely.
- Serve and enjoy.

Nutritional Value (Amount per Serving):

- Calories 192
- Fat 12.3 g
- Carbohydrates 19.4 g
- Sugar 8.6 g
- Protein 1.9 g
- Cholesterol 31 mg

THE "DIRTY DOZEN" AND "CLEAN 15"

The Environmental Working Group (EWG) publishes annual lists of produce containing the highest and lowest levels of pesticide residue. The lists are based on analyzing data from the USDA Pesticide Data Program report.

The EWG found that a majority (70%) of the 48 different kinds of produce tested contained some residue of at least one type of pesticide. Overall they found 178 different kinds of pesticides. This pesticide residue can remain on produce despite washing and peeling. Every kind of pesticide is toxic for people and ingesting them can cause damage to the immune system, reproductive system, nervous system, cancer, and more. Pregnant women may harm the health and development of the unborn baby as a result of consuming pesticide residue.

Keep these facts in mind when you are selecting produce and deciding whether to buy organic.

THE DIRTY DOZEN

- Celery
- Pears
- Spinach
- Strawberries
- Apples
- Nectarines
- Peaches
- Grapes
- Cherries
- Sweet bell peppers
- Tomatoes
- Potatoes

THE CLEAN 15

- Eggplant
- Cauliflower
- Sweet corn
- Pineapples
- Avocados
- Onions
- Cabbage
- Frozen sweet peas
- Asparagus
- Papayas
- Mangoes
- Honeydew
- Cantaloupe
- Kiwi
- Grapefruit

Measurement Conversion Tables

Volume Equivalents (Dry)

US Standard	Metric (Approx.)
¼ teaspoon	1 ml
½ teaspoon	2 ml
1 teaspoon	5 ml
1 tablespoon	15 ml
¼ cup	59 ml
½ cup	118 ml
1 cup	235 ml

Weight Equivalents

US Standard	Metric (Approx.)
½ ounce	15 g
1 ounce	30 g
2 ounces	60 g
4 ounces	115 g
8 ounces	225 g
12 ounces	340 g
16 oz or 1 lb	455 g

Volume Equivalents (Liquid)

US Standard	US Standard (ounces)	Metric (Approx.)
2 tablespoons	1 fl oz	30 ml
¼ cup	2 fl oz	60 ml
½ cup	4 fl oz	120 ml
1 cup	8 fl oz	240 ml
1 ½ cups	12 fl oz	355 ml
2 cups or 1 pint	16 fl oz	475 ml
4 cups or 1 quart	32 fl oz	1 L
1 gallon	128 fl oz	4 L

Oven Temperatures

Fahrenheit (F)	Celsius (C) (Approx)
250°F	120°C
300°F	150°C
325°F	165°C
350°F	180°C
375°F	190°C
400°F	200°C
425°F	220°C
450°F	230°C

References and Resources

Air-frying, pretreatment may decrease acrylamide in potatoes. (2015). *IFT*. Retrieved
19 April 2018, from
http://www.ift.org/food-technology/daily-news/2015/april/15/airfrying-pretreat
ment-may-decrease-acrylamide-in-potatoes.aspx

Best Air Frying Oil: Which Oil Should I Use With My Air Fryer?. *Air Cookers*. Retrieved
19 April 2018, from https://www.aircookers.com/cooking/air-fryer-oil/

Carla S.P. Santos, Lucía Molina-Garcia, Sara C. Cunha and Susana Casal, Fried potatoes:
Impact of prolonged frying in monounsaturated oils, *Food Chemistry*,
10.1016/j.foodchem.2017.09.117, 243,(192-201), (2018).
https://www.cancer.gov/about-cancer/causes-prevention/risk/diet/acrylamide-f
act-sheet

de Looper, C. (2018). Six Of The Best Air Fryers. Retrieved from
https://www.forbes.com/sites/forbes-finds/2018/06/24/best-air-fryers/

Ferreira FS, Sampaio GR, Keller LM, Sawaya ACHF, Chávez DWH, Torres EAFS,
Saldanha T.
(2017) *Impact of Air Frying on Cholesterol and Fatty Acids Oxidation in Sardines: Protective
Effects of Aromatic Herbs*.J Food Sci. 2017 Dec;82(12):2823-2831. doi: 10.1111/1750-
3841.13967.

Flores, J. (2018). *Top 10 Best Air Fryer Reviews and Buying Guide for 2018 -
Cookware Judge*. *Cookware Judge*. Retrieved 19 April 2018, from
http://www.cookwarejudge.com/top-10-best-air-fryer-reviews-buying-guide.html

Good, J. (2018). Healthiest Cooking Oil Comparison Chart with Smoke Points and
Omega 3 Fatty Acid Ratios. Retrieved from
https://jonbarron.org/diet-and-nutrition/healthiest-cooking-oil-chart-smoke-po
ints

Janeway, K. (2018). Countertop Air Fryers: More Than Hot Air?. Retrieved from
https://www.consumerreports.org/air-fryers/countertop-air-fryers-more-than-h
ot-air/

Knapp Rinella, H. (2017). *The Airfryer has a surprising number of uses. Las Vegas
Review-Journal*. Retrieved 19 April 2018, from
https://www.reviewjournal.com/entertainment/food/the-airfryer-has-a-surprising-number-
of-uses/

Krokida, M. K., Oreopolou, V. and Maroulis, Z. B. 2000. Water loss and oil uptake as a function of frying time. Journal of Food Engineering 44: 39–46.

Kumar, J., Das, S., & Teoh, S. (2018). Dietary Acrylamide and the Risks of Developing Cancer: Facts to Ponder. *Frontiers In Nutrition, 5*. doi: 10.3389/fnut.2018.00014

M. Arafat, S. (2014). Air Frying a New Technique for Produce of Healthy Fried Potato Strips. *Journal Of Food And Nutrition Sciences, 2*(4), 200. http://dx.doi.org/10.11648/j.jfns.20140204.26

Pelucchi, C., Bosetti, C., Galeone, C., & La Vecchia, C. (2014). Dietary acrylamide and cancer risk: An updated meta-analysis. *International Journal Of Cancer, 136*(12), 2912-2922. doi: 10.1002/ijc.29339

Praderio, C. (2015). *We Researched and Ranked 14 Cooking Oils. Which One Should You Buy?. Prevention*. Retrieved 19 April 2018, from https://www.prevention.com/eatclean/best-cooking-oils

Sansano, M., Juan-Borrás, M., Escriche, I., Andrés, A., & Heredia, A. (2015). Effect of Pretreatments and Air-Frying, a Novel Technology, on Acrylamide Generation in Fried Potatoes. *Journal Of Food Science, 80*(5), T1120-T1128. doi: 10.1111/1750-3841.12843

Shepherd, M. (2018). In Search Of Meteorology And Physics In Your Fancy New Air Fryer. Retrieved from https://www.forbes.com/sites/marshallshepherd/2017/12/27/in-search-of-meteorology-and-physics-in-your-fancy-new-air-fryer/#5142358c2005

Teruel, M., Gordon, M., Linares, M., Garrido, M., Ahromrit, A., & Niranjan, K. (2015). A Comparative Study of the Characteristics of French Fries Produced by Deep Fat Frying and Air Frying. *Journal Of Food Science, 80*(2), E349-E358. doi: 10.1111/1750-3841.12753

INDEX

Made in the USA
Middletown, DE
06 December 2018